MW00835331

Traeger Grill Bible Cookbook 2021: 2 BOOKS IN 1: The Ultimate Guide. Two Years of Delicious, Tasty, Quick & Easy Recipes for Advanced & Beginners

AUTHOR
John Brown
Steven Johnson

Traeger Grill: The Ultimate Guide: Smoker Cookbook & Wood Pellet with One Year of Quick & Easy Recipes for Beginners and Advanced

AUTHOR
John Brown

Contents

CHAPTER 1
Traeger Starters

What is Traeger Bible:

The Traeger is a wood pellet flame broil. In it, pellets are drawn from a side-mounted container into a focal consume chamber by a drill, at that point touched off by a hot metal pole. Those instruments run on power, so you must connect it. It offers exact, computerized temperature control incorporated with meat thermometers. To work it, you should simply fill the container with pellets, turn it on, and dial in whatever temperature you need—anything from "smoke" to 450 degrees Fahrenheit.

Conversely, the Big Green Egg is a carefully simple encounter. The Japanese Kamado-style flame broil is a major, egg-molded clay box that encourages definite temperature control by means of flexible wind current. Its shape and materials both appropriate warmth uniformly and hold in dampness. The Egg is more equipped for hitting both incredibly low temperatures (150-degree smokes are conceivable) and amazingly high ones than a common charcoal flame broil. My normal steak cooking strategy on it includes 1,200-degree burns. It's additionally fit for holding whatever temperature you need for expanded periods. Whenever you've begun it and balanced out the temperature, it's anything but difficult to set it at 200 degrees and leave for eight hours while your brisket smokes. It'll hold that temperature equally for that much time or more.

Honey Bourbon Wings:

Ingredients:

1) 2-1/2 pounds huge chicken wings

2) 1 12.8-ounce bottle Traeger Honey-Bourbon Barbecue Sauce, or your number one grill sauce

Method:

1) With a sharp blade, cut the wings into three pieces through the joints. Dispose of the wing tips, or put something aside for chicken stock. Move the leftover "drumettes" and "pads" to a huge resealable plastic pack.

2) Prepared to cook, start the Traeger flame broil on Smoke with the top open until the fire is set up (4 to 5 minutes). Set the gum-based paint true to 350 degrees F and preheat, top shut, for 10 to 15 minutes.

Jalapeno Poppers:

Ingredients:

1) 18 media to huge jalapeno peppers
2) 8 ounces cream cheddar, at room temperature
3) 4 ounces ground Mexican four-cheddar mix or cheddar
4) 1 teaspoon bean stew powder, or more to taste
5) 1/2 teaspoon garlic salt
6) 2 Scallions (green onions), managed, white and green parts minced
7) 8 to 10 cuts of slim cut bacon

Method:

1) Cut every jalapeno down the middle longwise

also, eliminate the ribs and seeds. An infant spoon or demitasse spoon functions admirably for this. (You may need to wear latex gloves.)

2) In a blending bowl, consolidate the cream cheddar, Mexican cheddar, stew powder, and garlic salt until very much mixed. Mix in the scallions. Move the combination to a quart-size resealable plastic sack. With a scissors, cut around 1/2-INCh off one of the lower corners to make a baked good pack. Press the cheddar blend into the jalapeno pepper parts. (Extra cheddar blend is magnificent on prepared potatoes.) Cut the bacon across into pieces adequately long to fold over the center of every jalapeno, crease side down. Orchestrate on a heating sheet covered with foil or material paper.

3) The bacon is cooked, and the cheddar is hot and foaming. Let cool for a couple of moments prior to serving.

Smoked Salmon:
Ingredients:

1) 1 Salmon filet (1-1/2 to 2 pounds), ideally wild-got
2) 1 Cup vodka or squeezed apple
3) 1 Cup earthy colored sugar or earthy colored sugar substitute, for example, SPLENDA
4) 1/2 Cup coarse (fit) salt
5) 1 tablespoon coarse dark pepper

Method:

1) Run your fingers over the salmon filet and eliminate any pin bones you find with kitchen tweezers or needle-nose pincers. Put the salmon filet in a huge resealable plastic pack and pour the vodka over it. Back rub the sack to ensure the salmon is submerged, at that point refrigerate for 1 to 2 hours.

2) Make the fix: Combine the sugar, salt, and dark pepper in another huge resealable plastic sack. Channel the fish. Dispose of the vodka. Add the filet to the sugar blend, ensuring the salmon is altogether covered. Refrigerate for 2 to 4 hours.

3) Rinse the fix off the salmon and dry with paper towels.

4) When prepared to cook, start the Traeger flame broil on Smoke with the cover open

until the fire is set up (4 to 5 minutes).

5) Arrange the salmon (skin-side down, on the off chance that it has skin) on the flame broil grind. (The specific time will rely upon the thickness of the filet.) There is no compelling reason to turn the fish. Utilizing a huge dainty spatula, move the salmon to a wire rack to cool. Cover the fish with saran wrap and refrigerate until spending time in jail.

Traeger Hot Smoked Trout:

Trout smoked on your Traeger and filled in as a hors d'oeuvre is ensured to dazzle supper visitors. It's stupendous when presented with salted onions on mixed drink breads, however can be "extended" by blending a cup of chipped smoked trout with 8 ounces of room temperature cream cheddar, 3 tablespoons of mollified spread, 1 tablespoon of new lemon squeeze, salt and pepper to taste.

Ingredients:

1) 1/2 Cup earthy colored sugar
2) 1/4 cup legitimate salt
3) 1 tablespoon pickling flavor
4) 1-quart

Method:

1) Make the saline solution: Combine the earthy colored sugar, salt, pickling zest, and water in a huge pitcher or canning container. Mix until the sugar and salt gems disintegrate. Open the trout. Run your fingers over the tissue to identify bones; eliminate any you find with kitchen tweezers or then again needle-nose pincers. Lower the trout in the salt water; refrigerate for 2 to 3 hours, however no more.

2) When prepared to cook, start the Traeger flame broil on Smoke with the top open until the fire is set up (4 to 5 minutes). Close the top.

3) Remove the trout from the salt water, knock off any enormous bits of the pickling flavors, and dry the fish on paper towels. Orchestrate the trout skin-side down on the flame broil grind.

4) Substance turns murky and chips effectively when nudged with a finger or fork. Move to a cooling rack. At the point when cool, cover with cling wrap and refrigerate until spending time in jail.

Chicken Quesadillas:

Dearest as an after-school-nibble, quesadillas are additionally an extraordinary method to commence a patio party! Collect these barbecue side and serve hot as your visitors show up. Forget about the chicken for a vegan choice.

Ingredients:

1) 4 10-INCh flour tortillas
2) Vegetable oil
3) 2 Cups ground Monterey Jack or pepper Jack cheddar
4) 2 Cups destroyed or cleaved cooked chicken (ideally made at a past barbecue meeting)
5) 1 small bundle new cilantro, leaves pulled off stems
6) 2 medium tomatoes, cultivated and diced
7) 4 scallions (green onions), managed, green and white parts meagerly cut
8) 1/4 cup cured jalapeno cuts, cleaved (discretionary)
9) Salt
10) Salsa or potentially acrid cream for serving

Method:

1) Lay a tortilla down on a rimmed heating sheet (or a huge bit of aluminum foil) covered gently with vegetable oil. Leave one-portion of the tortilla uncovered. Top the other half with a portion of the cheddar, chicken, cilantro leaves, tomatoes, scallions, and cured jalapenos, whenever wanted. Season with salt. Get done with somewhat more ground cheddar. (This will "stick" different fixings together as it softens.) Fold the exposed portion of the tortilla over the filled half and put in a safe spot. Rehash the cycle with the excess tortillas.

2) When prepared to cook, start the Traeger barbecue on Smoke with the cover open until the fire is set up (4 to 5 minutes). Set the gumbased to 375 degrees F and preheat, top shut, for 10 to 15 minutes.

3) With an enormous spatula, cautiously move the quesadillas to the flame broil grind. Cook until the cheddar is softened and the outside is starting to brown (8 to 10 minutes absolute). Utilizing the spatula, turn once part of the way through the cooking time. Cut every quesadilla into three wedges with a scissors or sharp blade. Present with salsa as well as sharp cream.

Teriyaki Wings:

Ingredients:

1) 2-1/2 pounds huge chicken wings
2) 1/2 Cup soy sauce
3) 1/4 cup water
4) 1/4 cup earthy colored
5) managed, white and green parts daintily cut
6) 1 Clove garlic, minced
7) 2 teaspoons sesame oil
8) 2 nickel-sized bits of new ginger, crushed
9) Vegetable oil for oiling the flame broil grind
10) 1 tablespoon sesame seeds, daintily toasted in a dry nonstick skillet

Method:

1) Dispose of the wing tips, or put something aside for chicken stock. Move the leftover "drumettes" and "pads" to an enormous resealable plastic pack or a bowl. In a little pot, consolidate the soy sauce, water, earthy colored sugar, vinegar, scallions, garlic, sesame oil, and ginger. Bring to a bubble, at that point decrease the warmth and stew for 10 minutes. Let cool totally, at that point pour over the chicken wings. Seal the sack and refrigerate for a few hours, or overnight. Channel the wings, disposing of the marinade.

2) When prepared to cook, start the Traeger flame broil on Smoke with the cover open

until the fire is set up (4 to 5 minutes). Set the gum based to 350 degrees F and preheat, cover shut, for 10 to 15 minutes. Oil the barbecue grind.

3) Arrange the wings on the flame broil grind. Turn once during the cooking time to keep the wings from adhering to the flame broil grind. Move to a platter or bowl and sprinkle with the sesame seeds.

Traeger Sausage Fatty:

Famous for quite a long while with grill and smoking lovers, "fatties" are typically 1-pound logs of smoked breakfast-type hotdog (now and again known as chubs). In addition to the fact that they are brilliant presented with eggs, bread rolls, or French toast, however when meagrely cut, they can twofold as canapés. A piece of ground espresso added to the rub echoes the morning meal subject. In case you're smoking one, you should smoke two. They'll vanish rapidly. Incidentally, when you cut the frankfurter, you'll see a dazzling pink smoke ring close to the surface a barbecue's "symbol of honour".

Ingredients:

1) 1 1-POUnd uncooked frankfurter chub, for example, Bob Evans or Jimmy Dignitary marks, any flavor
2) Traeger Pork and Poultry Rub, or your #1 grill rub
3) 1 tablespoon fine-to medium-pound espresso

Method:

1) Carefully eliminate the plastic wrapping from the frankfurter so the wiener remains log-molded, around 2-1/2 to 3 crawls in breadth. Season equitably with the Traeger Pork and Poultry Rub, at that point dust with the espresso.

2) When prepared to cook, start the Traeger

flame broil on Smoke with the top open until the fire is set up (4 to 5 minutes).

3) Smoke the wiener for 60 minutes. Increment the warmth to 225 degrees F. Keep on cooking the wiener until a moment read meat thermometer embedded through the end peruses 160 degrees F, around 45 minutes to 60 minutes.

Grilled Shrimp Cocktail:

Ingredients:

1) 1/4 cup extra-virgin olive oil
2) Traeger Veggie Shake, or your #1 grill rub
3) 1 Cup Traeger Chili Sauce, or your #1 stew sauce
4) 2 tablespoons arranged horseradish, or more to taste
5) 1 tablespoon new lemon or lime juice
6) 1 teaspoon Worcestershire sauce
7) A few drops of Tabasco sauce
8) Freshly ground dark pepper
9) Lemon wedges for serving
10) 6-inch bamboo sticks

Method:

1) In a medium bowl, throw the shrimp to cover with the olive oil and around 2 teaspoons of Traeger Veggie Shake. String the shrimp on the bamboo sticks, 2 to a stick. Consolidate

the stew sauce, horseradish, lemon juice, Worcestershire sauce, and Tabasco sauce in a little bowl, speeding to mix. Season to taste with pepper.

2) Arrange the shrimp sticks on the barbecue grind. Barbecue until firm and misty, 2 to 4 minutes for each side. Orchestrate on a plate or platter with the sauce and lemon wedges.

Barbecued Chicken Nachos:

Have you ever requested a plate of nachos in an eatery, just to find huge numbers of the chips passed up the fixings? Not exclusively is this formula a curve on customary variants, yet each chip conveys a payload of the multitude of fixings.

Ingredients:

1) 1-1/4 pounds boneless skinless chicken bosoms
2) Traeger Pork and Poultry Rub, or taco preparing
3) 24 enormous tortilla chips (not broken)
4) 3 cups (12 ounces) ground Mexican four-cheddar mix
5) 1/2 Cup cut dark olives, depleted
6) Sliced salted jalapenos (discretionary)
7) 3 scallions (green onions), managed, white and green parts meagerly cut

8) 1 Cup harsh cream, for serving

Method:

1) Leave the flame broil on in the event that you are making the nachos right away.

2) Dice the chicken into little 3D squares, 1/2-INCh or less. Move to a blending bowl and pour 1/2 Cup of Traeger Regular Barbecue Sauce over the diced chicken. Mix delicately to cover each piece. (Add more sauce if necessary, yet less that the combination is "gloppy".)

3) Lay the tortilla contributes a solitary layer on a rimmed preparing sheet or pizza dish. Sprinkle uniformly with a large portion of the cheddar. Spoon a tad bit of the grilled chicken combination on each chip. Top with dark olives and salted jalapeno, if wanted. Sprinkle the excess portion of the cheddar uniformly over the chips. Disperse the cut onions over the chips.

4) Put the preparing sheet on the flame broil grind. Prepare until the chips are fresh and the cheddar is dissolved, 12 to 15 minutes. With a spatula, move the nachos to a plate or platter. Serve promptly with the harsh cream.

Grilled Corn Salsa:

Salsa... it's not only for chips any longer. Flame broiled Corn Salsa is so adaptable, you can serve it over barbecued chicken, hamburger, or steak fish like fish, halibut, or swordfish. Or on the other hand pair it with flame broiled shrimp for an exceptional shrimp mixed drink. Change the salsa by adding diced red chime pepper or avocado, or a container of dark beans, washed and depleted.

Ingredients:

1) 4 tomatoes, for example, Roma, split
2) 1 medium-size onion, stripped and quartered through the root end
3) 1 teaspoon cumin
4) 1/4 cup new cilantro leaves, cleaved

Method:

1) Barbecue grind. Flame broil until the vegetables have pleasant singe blemishes on the cut sides. Flame broil the corn simultaneously, turning habitually, until a portion of the pieces are profoundly sautéed.

2) Blade, cut the corn pieces off the cob (on the off chance that you chip away at a clammy towel the portions won't dissipate to such an extent).

3) Move the barbecued vegetables to a blending

bowl. Mix in the garlic, vegetable oil, lime juice, Traeger Veggie Shake, cumin, furthermore, cilantro. Refrigerate any extras in a covered holder.

Pepperoni-Provolone Bread:

Ingredients:

1) 1 portion frozen bread mixture, for example, Rhodes
2) Extra-virgin olive oil
3) 1 teaspoon dried oregano
4) 1 teaspoon dried basil
5) 1 teaspoon dried parsley
6) 4 ounces meagerly cut pepperoni
7) 4 ounces meagerly cut provolone cheddar, or mozzarella
8) Cornmeal for tidying the preparing sheet

Method:

1) Defrost the bread mixture and let it rise ac floured kitchen counter or other level surface, fold and stretch the batter into a 12-by 18-inch square shape. (This takes a little tolerance if the mixture is extremely flexible. Brush with olive oil, and sprinkle uniformly with half of the oregano, basil, and parsley. Organize the pepperoni in a solitary layer on the batter, leaving a 1-INCh verge on all sides. Lay the cheddar on top of the pepperoni. Beginning the long side, roll the mixture up

uniformly jam move style. Squeeze the long crease together along its length. Squeeze the finishes together and fold under the portion, creasing the mixture to keep the cheddar and pepperoni encased.

2) Lay the bread, crease side down, on an oiled preparing sheet tidied daintily with cornmeal. Brush the top and favors olive oil, and sprinkle the leftover dried spices uniformly over it. Utilizing a bread blade, cut shallow vents in the top on a slanting. Cover with oiled cling wrap and let ascend in a warm spot for 30 minutes.

3) When prepared to cook, start the Traeger flame broil on Smoke with the top open until the fire is set up (4 to 5 minutes). Set the gum-based to 350 degrees F and preheat, cover shut, for 10 to 15 minutes.

4) Remove the cling wrap from the bread. Move the heating sheet with the bread to the flame broil. Bread is earthy colored and heated through. (It's smarter to overbake than underbake, for this situation.) Let the bread cool totally on a rack prior to cutting and serving.

CHAPTER 2
Traeger Beef

Beef Tips:

1) Marinate beef for the occasions coordinated by the formula. Don't over-marinate, or the meat can build up a soft surface.

2) For better shading and caramelization, thump the majority of the strong marinade fixings off meat (garlic, onions, and so forth) and dry it completely with paper towels prior to barbecuing.

3) Season beef not long prior to cooking with your number one Traeger Rub or Shake or salt and pepper. Something else, the salt will start to coax dampness out of the meat.

4) Always let beef rest prior to cutting or serving to permit the regular meat juices reallocate themselves; the time will rely upon the cut of meat. Let more slender steaks and cheeseburgers rest 2 to 3 minutes, thicker slices.

5) Keep meat refrigerated until you cook it. (The

"peril zone" is somewhere in the range of 40- and 140-degrees F.) Premium steakhouses never forget about their meats at room temperature.

6) Invest in a solid moment read or distant meat thermometer and remember cooking temperatures for uncommon (125 degrees F), medium-uncommon (135 to 140 degrees F), and all around done (150 degrees F or more).

7) Top steaks with a pat of room-temperature margarine prior to allowing them to rest for additional flavor and wealth.

8) Remember that meat will keep on rising a few degrees in temperature as it rests.

Barbecued Flat Iron Steaks:

A butcher trusted to us that level iron steaks (otherwise called beef shoul-der top edge steaks) are his number one cut of beef. Taken from the highest point of the hurl, they are substantial tasting, all around marbled, and are best when served medium-uncommon. Use them whenever you make fajitas.

Ingredients:

1) 4 level iron steaks, every 1/2-to 3/4-inch thick, 7 to 8 ounces each
2) Traeger Beef Rub, or your #1 grill rub
3) 2 tablespoons minced parsley

Method:

1) Season the steaks well on the two sides with Traeger Beef Rub. Focus on the flavoring with your fingers.

2) Arrange the steaks on the flame broil mesh and barbecue, turning once, for 8 to 10 minutes for medium-uncommon, or 11 to 13 minutes for medium, turning once part of the way through flame broiling. Move to a platter or plates and sprinkle with parsley. Let the steaks rest 2 minutes prior to serving to allow the juices to reallocate themselves.

Beef Tenderloin:

A two-venture cooking measure—burning and afterward simmering on the Traeger is probably the most ideal approaches to deal with this pricy, extraordinary event meat. You can streamline this formula by skirting the mustard covering, however it helps keep this lean cut clammy. A moment read meat thermometer will assist you with accomplishing the ideal level of doneness.

Ingredients:

1) 2 tablespoons extra-virgin olive oil (partitioned use)
2) 1 2-to 3-pound filet of beef, managed, ideally focus cut (see Note beneath)
3) 1/3 cup Dijon-style mustard
4) 1 teaspoon Worcestershire sauce

Method:

1) Heat a huge skillet, ideally cast iron, on the burner over medium-high warmth. Sparkling, placed the meat into the dish, singing it well on all sides. (Remember the closures: Carefully hold the meat upstanding with utensils.) Transfer the meat to a rimmed preparing sheet. In a little bowl, join the mustard, thyme, Worcestershire sauce, and the excess tablespoon of olive oil and blend well. Brush or slather the mustard blend over the outside of the filet.

2) When prepared to cook, start the Traeger flame broil on Smoke with the top open until the fire is set up (4 to 5 minutes).

3) Put the filet straightforwardly on the flame broil mesh and meal for 25 to 30 minutes, or until a moment read meat thermometer enrolls an inside temperature of 135 degrees F (for medium-uncommon). Cook less time in the event that you favor your meat more extraordinary than that, or additional time in the event that you like it very much done. Move to a cutting board and let the meat rest, risen with aluminum foil, for 5 minutes prior to cutting and serving.

Traeger Smoked T-Bones:

A T-bone (and its bigger cousin, the Porterhouse) comprises of a strip steak and a tenderloin isolated by a T-moulded bone. Finishing off the meat with margarine is a stunt utilized by extravagant steakhouses.

Ingredients:

1) 4 T-bone steaks (14-to 16-OUnces each), at any rate 1-INCh thick
2) Your most loved Traeger Rub, or coarse salt and newly ground dark pepper
3) 4 tablespoons margarine, at room temperature

Method:

1) Season the steaks on the two sides with the Traeger Rub.

2) When prepared to cook, start the Traeger barbecue on Smoke with the top open until the fire is set up (4 to 5 minutes).

3) Arrange the steaks on the barbecue mesh and smoke for 30 minutes.

Better Burgers:

As of late, we've been tested to cook beef burgers to a safe inward temperature of 160 degrees F without drying them out. That is a troublesome request on a regular flame broil, yet simple on a Traeger. The delicate backhanded warmth cooks the meat through and leaves it delicious as can be.

Ingredients:

1) 2 pounds ground throw, 80/20 or 85/15 (shelter fat proportion)
2) 3 tablespoons spread, liquefied
3) 4 Kaiser moves, part
4) Lettuce leaves
5) Sweet onion cuts
6) Tomato cuts
7) Dill pickle chips

Method:

1) Make sure the meat is very much chilled prior to taking care of. Consolidate the ground beef and Traeger Beef Rub in a medium bowl. Wet your hands with cold water, and blend delicately. Separation the meat into four equivalent bits. Rewet your hands with cold water, and structure each segment into a patty around 4 crawls in breadth and 3/4-inch thick. (Make an effort not to exhaust the meat.) Using your thumbs, make a shallow wide sadness on the highest point of every burger. (This keeps the burger from building up a lump in the center.)

2) Combine the mayonnaise and the grill sauce in a shallow bowl and refrigerate until spending time in jail.

3) Brush the cut sides of the Kaiser moves with the dissolved margarine.

4) When prepared to cook, start the Traeger flame broil on Smoke with the top open until the fire is set up.

5) Arrange the burgers straightforwardly on the barbecue grind, sadness side down. Cook for 10 minutes, at that point moment read meat thermometer

6) Meanwhile, daintily toast the buns, chopped sides down. Watch cautiously as buttered bread can undoubtedly consume.

7) Puta burger on every bun base, and top with lettuce, onion, tomato, and pickle. Get done with the highest point of the bun. Serve right away.

Horseradish Cream:

Prime rib is, obviously, one of the most extravagant cuts of beef you can purchase. Furthermore, it's astounding when simmered on a Traeger. A far-off meat thermometer is a genuine assistance when cooking an enormous, bone-in dish like prime rib. It will take out the need to lift the flame broil top as often as possible to keep an eye on your speculation. Recollect that the meal will keep on cooking as it rests, so take it off the flame broil when it is 5 to 10 degrees cooler than your ideal serving temperature.

Ingredients:

1) One 3-to-4-pound prime rib
2) Traeger Prime Rib or Beef Rub, or equivalent pieces of legitimate salt and coarsely ground dark pepper
3) Granulated garlic (discretionary)
4) Horseradish Cream (formula follows)
5) Large simmering skillet with a meat rack
6) Butcher's string

Method:

1) Bind it at stretches with butcher's string. (This shields it from isolating along the internal fat line as it cooks.) Season the meal well with the Traeger Prime Rib or Beef Rub, or the salt pepper blend. Sprinkle with the granulated garlic, whenever wanted. Utilize your fingers to pat the flavors into the meat. Spot the meat rack in the broiling skillet; put the meal, bone-side down and revealed, on the rack.

2) When prepared to cook, start the Traeger flame broil on Smoke with the top open until the fire is set up.

3) Roast for 30 minutes. Lessen the temperature to 300 degrees F, and keep on cooking until the inward temperature in the thickest piece of the meat peruses 130 degrees F (for medium-uncommon) as perused on a moment read meat thermometer.

4) Eliminate the butcher's string. Move the meat to a huge cutting board. With a sharp blade, cut off the rack of bones and set them aside for chewing. Cut the meat and serve quickly with the Horseradish Cream (see underneath).

Brisket is a cut from between a cow's forelegs. It is a muscle utilized habitually by the creature, which clarifies its beefy flavour and its should be cooked low and delayed for quite a long time. Search for a brisket with a cap of fat in any event 1/4-inch thick. Permit additional time than you might suspect you'll require as each brisket is extraordinary. What's more, continually carry it to an inside temperature of 190 to 195 degrees F for greatest delicacy. Prepared beans are an extraordinary backup.

Ingredients:

1) 1 6-pound brisket level, managed
2) Traeger Beef Rub, or your #1 grill rub
3) 2 Cups beef stock, lager, or cola
4) 1/4 cup apple juice vinegar
5) 2 tablespoons Worcestershire sauce
6) Traeger Texas Spicy Barbecue Sauce, or your #1 grill sauce

Method:

1) Season the brisket on the two sides with the Traeger Beef Rub. Make the mop sauce: In a perfect shower bottle, join the beef stock, lager, or cola with the vinegar and Worcestershire sauce.

2) When prepared to cook, start the Traeger barbecue on Smoke with the top open until the fire is set up (4 to 5 minutes). Orchestrate the brisket fat-side up on the barbecue grind and smoke for 3 to 4 hours, showering with the

mop sauce each keep on cooking the brisket, showering incidentally with mop sauce, until a moment read thermometer embedded in the thickest piece of the meat peruses 190 to 195 degrees F. (This will probably take 4 to 6 hours more, or much more. Be patient and don't surge the cycle.)

3) Ideally in a protected compartment fixed with thick shower towels or papers so the meat remains hot. Cut with a sharp blade across the grain into pencil-width cuts. Serve the grill sauce independently as an afterthought.

Barbecued Brisket:

Brisket is one intense cut of meat. Most importantly, it requires tolerance with respect to the barbecue. It might require some investment to get from 150 degrees F to 190 degrees F, a period known as a "level". Try not to be enticed to turn the warmth up now. On the off chance that your brisket is delicate before your visitors show up, wrap it firmly in foil, at that point thick towels and let it rest in a protected cooler. It will remain hot for over 60 minutes. You can likewise rewarm foil-wrapped brisket on your Traeger or in your stove (275 to 300 degrees F).

Ingredients:
1) 2 tablespoons earthy colored sugar
2) 1 tablespoon chile powder
3) 1 teaspoon garlic salt
4) 1/4 cup Traeger Prime Rib Rub
5) 1 tablespoon ground espresso
6) 1 4-to 5-pound focus cut brisket level, managed
7) Traeger Texas Spicy Barbecue Sauce
8) 9x13-inch aluminum foil dispensable container
9) Aluminum foil
10) A clean splash bottles
11) Cup cold blended espresso

Method:

1) Make the mop sauce: Combine the espresso, lager, earthy colored sugar, chile powder and garlic salt in a bowl and race to break down any salt or sugar precious stones. Move to a perfect shower jug and put in a safe spot.

2) In a little bowl, blend the Traeger Prime Rib Rub and the ground espresso. Rub this combination on the brisket, covering all surfaces.

3) When prepared to cook, start the Traeger barbecue on Smoke with the top open until the fire is set up (4 to 5 minutes).

4) Put the brisket straightforwardly on the barbecue mesh and smoke for 2 hours. Shower the brisket with the mop sauce and move to a dispensable aluminum foil dish. Increment the temperature to 275 degrees F and keep on cooking for 4 to 5 hours, splashing each hour with the mop sauce. In the event that anytime the brisket seems, by all accounts, to be drying out, cover it firmly with aluminum foil. (Stop cleaning in the event that you do this.) When done, the interior temperature of the brisket will be 185 to 190 degrees F (anything less, and your brisket will be intense). Serve, whenever wanted, with grill sauce as an afterthought. Great backups incorporate heated beans and rolls or cornbread.

5) Note: "Grain"— the heading the long meat filaments run—can be hard to follow in a brisket.

Beef Brisket:

Whenever you've tasted corned beef cooked in its own juices on your Traeger, you'll never return to bubbled corned beef again. What's more, extras, in the event that you have any, make fantastic Reuben sandwiches.

Ingredients:

1) 1 Corned beef brisket level, 3 to 4 pounds
2) 1/4 cup Dijon-style mustard

Method:

1) Eliminate the corned beef brisket from its bundling and dispose of the flavor parcel, assuming any.

2) When prepared to cook, start the Traeger barbecue on Smoke with the top open until the fire is set up.

3) Put the corned beef brisket straightforwardly on the flame broil grind, fat side up, and cook for 2 hours. In the interim, join the grill sauce and the mustard in a medium bowl, racing to blend.

4) Pour half of the grill sauce-mustard blend in the lower part of an expendable aluminum foil skillet. With utensils, move the brisket to the skillet, fat-side up. Pour the rest of the grill sauce-mustard combination over the highest point of the brisket, utilizing a spatula to spread the sauce uniformly. Cover the container firmly with aluminum foil. Return the brisket to the flame broil and keep on cooking for 2 to 3 hours, or until the brisket is delicate. The interior temperature should be 185 degrees F on a moment read meat thermometer. Permit the meat to rest for 15 to

20 minutes.

5) Slice across the grain into 1/4-INCh cuts with a sharp blade and serve right away. Whenever wanted, spoon a portion of the sauce over each serving.

Beef Jerky:

Make certain to cut back out any excess or connective tissue you see when you're setting up the meat. Since some dampness will be left in the jerky toward the finish of the smoking time, refrigerate the meat for longer-term stockpiling.

Ingredients:

1) 1/2 Cup soy sauce
2) 1/2 Cup lager, cola, or water
3) 1/4 cup Worcestershire sauce
4) 2 teaspoons garlic powder
5) 1 teaspoon onion powder
6) 1 teaspoon newly ground dark pepper
7) 2 pounds managed beef top or base round, sirloin tip, or flank steak

Method:

1) In a blending bowl, join the soy sauce, water, Worcestershire sauce, garlic powder, onion powder, and pepper and speed to blend.

2) With a sharp blade, cut the beef into 1/4-inch-thick cuts contrary to what would be expected. (This is simpler if the meat is somewhat frozen.) Trim any fat or connective tissue. Put the beef cuts in an enormous resealable plastic pack. Pour the soy sauce combination over the beef, and back rub the sack so all the cuts get covered with the marinade. Seal the pack and refrigerate for a few hours, or overnight.

3) When prepared to cook, start the Traeger barbecue on Smoke with the top open until the fire is set up (4 to 5 minutes).

4) Remove the beef from the marinade and dispose of the marinade. Dry the beef cuts between paper towels. Mastermind the meat in a solitary layer straightforwardly on the flame broil grind.

5) Move to a resealable plastic sack while the jerky's actually warm. Allow the jerky to rest for an hour at room temperature. Press any air from the sack, and refrigerate the jerky. It will save for half a month.

Filets Mignons:

Cut from the little finish of an entire beef tenderloin, filets mignons are ideal for a supper for two. Attempt to purchase steaks that are at any rate an inch thick on the off chance that you favour your filets uncommon or medium-uncommon. Despite the fact that it's discretionary, you can fold a piece of bacon over the outside of each filet prior to cooking for a fancier introduction. Mushrooms sautéed with margarine, garlic, and a sprinkle of Worcestershire sauce make a decent side dish.

Method:

1) When prepared to cook, start the Traeger flame broil on Smoke with the cover open until the fire is set up.

2) Arrange the steaks on the barbecue grind. Cook for 7 minutes. Turn with utensils, and cook for 5 to 7 minutes more, or until the interior temperature arrives at 135 degrees F on a moment read meat thermometer embedded through the side toward the focal point of the steak. (Change the time on the off chance that you incline toward your meat all the more all around done.)

Flank Steak:

Serious exercise, giving it extraordinary flavour. In any case, except if it's appropriately cooked and cut, it very well may be an extreme bite. Afterward cut it daintily on a corner to corner across the grain. Extras make fantastic sandwiches.

Method:

1) In a little bowl, whisk together the oil, vinegar, and mustard.

2) Lay the flank steak in a preparing dish sufficiently huge to hold it. Season the flank steak on the two sides with the Traeger Beef Rub, tapping the flavoring down with your fingertips.

3) Pour the oil blend over it, going to cover, at that point top with the onions and garlic. Marinate, covered with saran wrap and refrigerated, for 4 to 8 hours, turning once.

4) When prepared to cook, start the Traeger flame broil on Smoke with the top open until the fire is set up.

5) Lift the flank steak from the marinade (dispose of the marinade and solids) and wipe off with paper towels. Mastermind the steak at a corner to corner straightforwardly on the flame broil grind. Flame broil for 6 minutes, at

that point turn. Keep flame broiling for 6 to 8 minutes more. (The specific time will rely upon the thickness of your steak.) Transfer the steak to a cutting load up and let rest for 5 minutes. Preseason with Traeger Beef Rub, whenever wanted. Cut daintily on the askew across the grain. Serve right away.

London Broil:

Meat all around done, this isn't the formula for you. London Broil is best served uncommon to medium-uncommon. Incidentally, London Broil is anything but a specific cut of meat—rather, it is a cooking strategy. The meat itself can be a few things, including top round, throw steak, flank steak, or even beef tenderloin.

Method:

1) Enormous resealable plastic pack. Go to cover. Refrigerate for a few hours, or overnight.

2) When prepared to cook, start the Traeger flame broil on Smoke with the top open until the fire is set up.

3) Remove the meat from the marinade. Whenever wanted, pour the marinade in a little pot and heat to the point of boiling over high warmth. Bubble for two minutes, at that point eliminate from the warmth. Strain, and

let cool. Presently you can utilize the marinade as a sauce. Keep warm.

4) Pat the meat dry with paper towels. Put the meat on the barbecue mesh and flame broil 8 to 10 minutes for every side, turning once with utensils, or until a moment read meat thermometer embedded into the thickest part peruses 135 degrees F for uncommon. (Barbecue a couple of moments longer in the event that you incline toward your London Broil medium-uncommon.) Let the meat rest for 3 minutes prior to cutting meagrely on a slanting contrary to what would be expected. Serve the warmed marinade as a sauce, whenever wanted.

Traeger Beef Roast:

Much the same as Mom used to make if Mom had a Traeger! Don't hesitate to cook potatoes, carrots, and onions close by the meal whenever wanted. Chill any left-overs, cut daintily, and use to develop sandwiches.

Method:

1) Rub the meal on all sides with the oil and spot on a rack in a simmering skillet, fat-side up. Season well with the Traeger Beef Shake. Pour the beef stock in the lower part of the skillet.

2) When prepared to cook, start the Traeger barbecue on Smoke with the top open until the fire is set up.

3) Cook the meal for 25 to 30 minutes, or until the outside is singed. Lessen the temperature to 225 degrees F and keep cooking, 2 to 3 hours, or until medium-uncommon (135 degrees F on a moment read meat thermometer). Allow it to arrive at 155 degrees F on the off chance that you favor your meat all around done. Tent the meal with aluminum foil and let the meat rest for 10 minutes prior cutting across the grain into slender cuts. Serve with the container drippings, whenever wanted.

Beef ribs:

Substantial beef long bones—likewise got back to beef ribs, save ribs, or Texas ribs—can be hard to track down. Butchers typically trim the meat as near the bone as conceivable to expand the poundage of boneless prime rib broil or potentially rib-eye steaks they can sell. So, whenever you overdo it on a prime rib broil, request that the butcher split the distinction by leaving more meat on the bones. (At times, they'll do this regardless of whether you don't accept the entire prime rib!) These ribs are not to be mistaken for beef toss ribs, likewise called "dinosaur" bones.

Ingredients:

1) Traeger Prime Rib Rub, or your number one grill rub
2) Traeger Texas Spicy Barbecue Sauce, or your number one grill sauce

Method:

1) On the off chance that your butcher has not effectively done as such, eliminate the flimsy papery layer from the bone-side of the ribs by working the tip of a spread blade or a screwdriver under the film over a center bone. Use paper towels to get a strong grasp, at that point detach the layer.

2) Whenever wanted, wrap the ribs firmly in foil partially through the cooking time. The most recent 30 minutes, cautiously eliminate the ribs from the foil and brush them generously with Traeger Texas Spicy Barbecue Sauce, and re-visitation of flame broil.

Santa Maria-Style Tri-Tip:

Up to this point, barely any individuals outside the Santa Maria Valley in Central California knew about tri-tip, a three-sided muscle from the lower part of the sirloin. Yet, its beefy flavour is getting on in different pieces of the nation. In some cases, you'll see it cut into steaks. It is generally served medium-uncommon with new salsa, pinquito beans, French bread, and a green serving of mixed greens.

Ingredients:

1) 1 tri-tip cook
2) Dark pepper, and garlic powder

Method:

1) 1-1/2 teaspoons each salt, newly ground dark pepper, and garlic powder Traeger Beef Rub.

2) When prepared to cook, start the Traeger barbecue on Smoke with the top open until the fire is set up.

3) Lay the tri-tip straightforwardly on the barbecue mesh and cook for 45 to 50 minutes. (Try not to overcook or the tri-tip with be extreme.

Chili-Glazed Meatloaf:

Meatloaf makes an extraordinary Sunday night dinner. (Ideally, you'll have extras for Monday sandwiches.) A line of cleaved entire carrots in the portion dish acts like a characteristic meat rack and shields the lower part of the meatloaf from getting dry.

Ingredients:

1) 1-1/2 pounds ground beef
2) 1/2-pound ground pork
3) 1 Cup dried bread scraps
4) 1/4 cup finely minced onion
5) 1 tablespoon Traeger Cajun Rub, or your number one grill rub
6) 1 teaspoon garlic powder
7) 2 eggs
8) 1/2 Cup milk
9) 2 teaspoons Worcestershire sauce
10) 2 whole carrots, stripped, managed, cut into lengths the width of your portion dish

Method:

1) In a huge blending bowl, join the ground beef, ground pork, bread scraps, onion, Traeger Cajun Rub, and the garlic powder. In another bowl, beat the eggs softly.

2) Add milk and Worcestershire sauce. Add the fluid fixings to the meat combination, and blend in with your hands. Lay a couple of the carrot pieces down in the portion container; the carrots will turn into a characteristic rack for the meat. Structure the meat into a portion shape and lay it on top of the carrots.

3) Put the portion skillet on the flame broil rack. Prepare the meatloaf for 50 to an hour, or until the inner temperature peruses 160 degrees F when perused on a moment read most recent 10 minutes of cooking. Move the meatloaf to a cooling rack and let cool for 10 minutes. Cautiously eliminate it from the portion skillet. (Dispose of the carrots.) Slice into 1/2-INCh cuts for serving.

Chimichurri Sauce:

Beef shoulder tenders are a reasonable option in contrast to pricy beef tenderloin. Additionally called "butcher's steak"— which gives you a sign of how great this slice is since butchers used to save it for themselves—this long, thin muscle from the shoulder toss is both fit and beefy-tasting. In the underneath readiness, the meat is prepared essentially, at that point barbecued over high warmth until medium-uncommon—similarly as they would do it in South America—and presented with chimichurri sauce, once in a while alluded to as "Argentinean steak sauce."

Ingredients:

1) 1/4 cup new parsley leaves, coarsely cleaved
2) 3 cloves garlic, coarsely cleaved
3) 2 teaspoons dried oregano
4) 1 teaspoon dried red pepper pieces, or more to taste
5) 1/4 cup red wine vinegar
6) 1/2 Cup extra-virgin olive oil

Method:

1) Season the shoulder tenders with Traeger

2) Make the chimichurri: In a blender container or little food processor, join the parsley, garlic, oregano, dried red pepper pieces, and red wine vinegar. Heartbeat until mixed. Add salt and pepper to taste. Allow the blend to sit

for 20 minutes for the flavors to create. At that point gradually mix in the olive oil.

3) When prepared to cook, start the Traeger barbecue on Smoke with the cover open until the fire is set up.
4) Arrange the shoulder tenders on the flame broil grind. Turn following 10 minutes to put barbecue marks on the opposite side. Barbecue to the ideal level of doneness, 5 to 10 minutes more for medium-uncommon (135 degrees F on a moment read meat thermometer).

5) Cut it on a corner to corner into cuts 3/4-inch thick. Whenever wanted, pour a portion of the chimichurri over the meat and serve the remainder of the sauce as an afterthought. Or on the other hand serve the sauce independently.

Southwestern Pot Roast:

Braised until it's self-destructing delicate, you can serve this over rice or in a tortilla or taco shells.

Ingredients:

1) 1 3-to 4-pound boneless throw cook
2) Traeger Fajita Rub, or salt and newly ground dark pepper
3) 2 tablespoons oil
4) 1 huge onion, stripped and coarsely slashed

5) 2 Cloves garlic, minced
6) 1 Cup beef stock
7) 1 10-ounce can dice tomatoes with green chiles
8) 1 teaspoon cumin

Method:

1) Heat an enormous skillet over medium-high warmth.

2) Add the oil. At the point when the oil sparkles, burn the meal on all sides. Move the meal to a lidded meal or heating dish adequately enormous to hold it. Diminish the warmth to medium and add the onions, mixing once in a while.

3) Add the beef stock, blending to scrape up the earthy colored pieces from the lower part of the container. At that point add the tomatoes, chile powder, oregano, and cumin and bring to a stew. Add salt and pepper to taste. Tip the onion-tomato blend over the meat. Put the cover on the meal. In the event that utilizing a preparing dish, cover it firmly with aluminum foil.

4) When prepared to cook, start the Traeger flame broil on Smoke with the cover open until the fire is set up (4 to 5 minutes).

5) Put the meal or container on the flame broil grind. Broil until the meat is exceptionally delicate, 3 to 4 hours. (Be cautious while

lifting the goulash top or foil as steam will get away.) Slice and present with the tomato-onion sauce.

Beef Short Ribs:

Traeger Chili Sauce joined with root lager and onions makes a delightful braising sauce for beef short ribs.

Ingredients:

1) 1 Cup great quality root lager pop, for example, Dr. Earthy colored's or Hanne's, in addition to additional case by case
2) 1 tablespoon new thyme leaves, slashed
3) 1 enormous sweet onion, meagerly cut into rings
4) 3 to 4 pounds bone-in short ribs, or 2-1/2 pounds of boneless short ribs
5) Salt
6) Freshly ground dark pepper
7) A 9x13-inch aluminum foil dispensable heating skillet or other preparing dish
8) Aluminum foil

Method:

1) Arrange the onions equitably in the lower part of the container. Pour the stew root brew sauce equitably over the ribs. Cover the container firmly with aluminum foil.

2) When prepared to cook, start the Traeger

flame broil on Smoke with the cover open until the fire is set up.

3) Put the dish of ribs on the flame broil mesh and cook for 2-1/2 to 3 hours, or until the ribs are delicate however not tumbling off the bone. Add a smidgen more root brew to the container if the dish doesn't appear to be sassy enough. Serve right away with polenta or pureed potatoes. Short ribs render a considerable lot of fat, so in the event that it concerns you, refrigerate the ribs in the sauce for the time being. The fat will have set on top, and can be taken out and disposed of prior to warming the ribs.

Korean Barbecued Short Ribs:

Crosscut beef short ribs, don't hesitate to substitute another cut of beef, for example, sirloin or toss, cut 1/4-inch thick across the grain. The marinade is likewise great on rib-eyes, skirt steak, and even chicken thighs or bosoms.

Ingredients:

1) 1/2 Cup soy sauce
2) 1/2 Cup water
3) 2 tablespoons white vinegar or rice vinegar
4) 2 tablespoons earthy colored sugar
5) 1 tablespoon granulated sugar or honey
6) 2 Cloves garlic, minced
7) 1 ready pear, stripped, cored, and coarsely hacked
8) 1 1-INCh piece new ginger, stripped and cut into coins
9) 1 Scallion (green onion), managed and coarsely slashed
10) 2 teaspoons sesame oil
11) 1 teaspoon Traeger Beef Shake, or salt

Method:

1) Lay the beef in a solitary layer in a heating dish and season on both sides with Traeger Beef Shake. Pour the marinade over the beef, surrendering the beef to cover the two sides. Cover and refrigerate for a few hours, or overnight.

2) When prepared to cook, start the Traeger barbecue on Smoke with the cover open until the fire is set up.

3) Remove the beef from the marinade; dispose of marinade. Mastermind the beef on the flame broil mesh and barbecue, 2 to 3 minutes for every side, or until the meat is cooked however you would prefer. (In Korea, they favor their short ribs very much done.)

Italian Meatball Subs:

These sandwiches are for good cravings—ideal for game day or a bustling weeknight dinner. You can likewise shape the meat combination into mixed drink size meatballs (utilize smaller than expected biscuit tins to heat them for roughly 20 minutes) and serve on toothpicks with warm marinara as a plunging sauce.

Ingredients:

1) 1-1/2 pounds ground beef
2) 1/2-pound mass Italian hotdog or ground pork
3) 3/4 cup prepared dry bread scraps
4) 1/2 Cup ground Parmesan
5) 1/4 cup onion, finely minced
6) 2 Cloves garlic, finely minced
7) 1 egg, daintily
8) Your most loved jolted spaghetti or marinara sauce
9) 4 hoagie or sub moves, split through the side

CHAPTER 3
Traeger Pork

Pork Tips:

1) Generally, bone-in meat will have more flavor than boneless cuts.

2) Always eliminate the slight layer on the rear of a rack of ribs to build smoke and zest assimilation. (Utilize the tip of a screwdriver or margarine blade to get under the film, at that point grasp.

3) For additional flavor, wrap fewer fatty cuts of pork, (for example, tenderloin or pork midsection broil) with cuts of bacon while cooking.

4) Tuck a container of squeezed apple into a side of the Traeger to keep meat soggy during long cooks (particularly great with ribs). On the other hand, move the juice to a spotless splash bottle and intermittently fog the meat. Recollect that lifting the top will add to your absolute cooking time.

5) Like poultry, pork at times profits by tenderizing prior to cooking.

6) Apply grill sauce the most recent couple of minutes of cooking to "set" the sauce and evade searing it. (Most sauces are high in sugars, which tend to consume on the flame broil.)

7) A pinkish ring just beneath the outside of the meat (and now and then on the bone also) is known as a "smoke ring," and is the indication of a smoking position all around done!

8) If flame broiling slashes rimmed with a layer of fat, make little vertical slices in the fat to deter it from twisting as the hacks cook.

Baby Back Ribs:

The 3-2-1 technique for grilling ribs—3 hours of smoke, 2 hours wrapped firmly in foil, and 1 hour sauced—has gotten extremely famous among rivalry barbecues and home cooks the same, particularly the individuals who incline toward their ribs "tumble off-the-bone" delicate. Change the cooking time in the event that you like your ribs with more bite. Don't hesitate to substitute extra ribs in this formula: They'll set aside a similar measure of effort to cook.

Ingredients:

1) 2 racks infant back pork ribs (around 5 pounds all out), managed
2) 1/3 cup yellow mustard
3) 1/2 Cup squeezed apple (isolated use), in addition to more if necessary

4) 1 tablespoon Worcestershire sauce
5) Traeger Pork and Poultry Rub, or your #1 grill rub
6) 1/2 Cup stuffed dull earthy colored sugar
7) 1/3 cup honey, warmed
8) Traeger BBQ Sauce, or your #1 grill sauce

Method:

1) If your butcher has not effectively done as such, eliminate the flimsy papery layer margarine blade or a screwdriver under the film over a center bone. Use paper towels to get a strong hold, at that point remove the layer.

2) In a little bowl, join the mustard, 1/4 cup of squeezed apple (hold the rest), and the Worcestershire sauce. Spread meagerly on the two sides of the ribs; season with Traeger Pork and Poultry Rub.

3) Move the ribs to a rimmed heating sheet however leave the flame broil on. Set the temperature to 225 degrees F.

4) Tear off four long sheets of hard core aluminium foil. Sprinkle a large portion of the earthy coloured sugar on the rack, at that point top with a large portion of the honey and half of the leftover squeezed apple. (Utilize somewhat more apple juice in the event that you need.) Lay another bit of foil on top and firmly crease the edges so there's no spillage.

Rehash with the excess rack of ribs.

5) Return the thwarted ribs to the flame broil and cook for an extra 2 hours. Cautiously eliminate the foil from the ribs—look out for hot steam—and brush the ribs on the two sides with Traeger BBQ Sauce. Dispose of the foil. Mastermind the ribs straightforwardly on the flame broil mesh and keep on barbecuing until the sauce "fixes", 30 minutes to 1 hour more. Allow the ribs to rest for a couple of moments prior to serving.

Memphis-Style Baby Back Ribs:

They like their ribs sassy and cooked low and delayed in Kansas City and different spots, however not in Memphis: There, the ribs are flame broiled straightforwardly over the warmth, are prepared in the wake of barbecuing, and are served sans grill sauce. Cooking time on these child backs is simply 2 to 3 hours—a fraction of the hour of expectedly grilled ribs—settling on them a decent decision for occupied days or evenings.

Ingredients:

1) 2 racks infant back pork ribs (around 5 pounds

absolute), managed

2) Traeger Pork and Poultry Rub, or your #1 grill rub

3) 2 Cups squeezed apple in a portion container or pie plate, in addition to more if necessary

Method:

1) In the event that your butcher has not effectively done as such, eliminate the flimsy papery film from the bone-side of the ribs by working the tip of a margarine blade or a screwdriver under the film over a center bone. Use paper towels to get a solid hold, at that point tear the layer off.

2) Put the squeezed apple in a side of the barbecue grind.

3) Arrange the ribs on the barbecue grind, meat-side up. Cook for 2 hours. Check the ribs. They should be pleasantly cooked and destroy effectively in your fingers.

4) If they're not done however you would prefer, return them to the barbecue, checking them like clockwork. Renew the squeezed apple if necessary.

5) When the ribs are done, move them toa cutting board and season them with Traeger Pork and Poultry Rub. Allow them to rest for a few moments prior to cutting into half chunks or individual ribs.

Pork Loin Roast:

Despite the fact that customary in numerous families for New Year's Day, pork flank broil is a conservative decision any season. For a certain something, there's practically no waste; and for another, it's regularly at a bargain. Locate the plastic packs of sauerkraut frequently sold in the meat division or refrigerated segment of stores. Feel free, however, to substitute canned sauerkraut.

Ingredients:

1) 1 1-POUnd sack of refrigerated sauerkraut
2) 2 Cooking apples, (for example, Granny Smith), cored and hacked
3) 1/3 cup earthy colored sugar
4) 1 pork midsection broil, 2 to 2-1/2 pounds
5) Traeger Sweet Rub, or salt and pepper

Method:

1) Lower part of a 9-by 13-inch glass preparing dish. Sprinkle equally with the earthy colored sugar. Season the pork cook with Traeger Sweet Rub and lay it on top of the sauerkraut-apple blend, fat-side up.

2) When prepared to cook, start the Traeger flame broil on Smoke with the cover open until the fire is set up (4 to 5 minutes). Set the temperature to 350 degrees F.

3) In the interim, mix the sauerkraut-apple combination and organize it on a platter. Cut the pork dish and shingle the cuts on top of the sauerkraut and apples. Serve right away.

Pork Shoulder Steaks:

Pork shoulder steaks—likewise called edge steaks—are regularly an incentive at the meat counter. In the event that you purchase steaks that are more slender than one inch, prior to cooking to deter them from twisting.

Ingredients:

1) 4 pork shoulder steaks, 1-to 1-1/4-INCh thick
2) Traeger Pork and Poultry Rub, or your #1 rub
3) 1 Cup Traeger Honey-Bourbon Barbecue Sauce, or your number one grill sauce

Method:

1) Prepared to cook, start the Traeger flame broil on Smoke with the top open until the fire is set up (4 to 5 minutes).
2) Grill the stakes for 35 to 40 minutes, or until they arrive at 160 degrees F on a moment read meat thermometer. The most recent 15 minutes, brush every steak on the two sides with the Traeger Honey-Bourbon Barbecue Sauce. Let the steaks rest for 3 minutes prior to serving.

Stuffed Pork Chops:

They rarely show up on American tables nowadays, yet stuffed pork cleaves merit a rebound: delicate, delicious pork slashes with an exquisite dressing that gets flavourfully crunchy outwardly. Prepared apples, put on the Trae-ger when you start the cleaves, make a fine pastry.

Ingredients:

1) 4 thick-cut (1-INCh) pork flank slashes, ideally with pockets cut in each
2) 2 Cups spice prepared or cornbread stuffing blend, for example, Pepperidge Farm

Method:

1) If your butcher has not effectively done as such, cut a profound pocket in the side of each hack with a little sharp blade, cutting toward the bone, however, not completely through.

2) Prepare the stuffing blend as per the bundle bearings, adding your own contacts whenever wanted (hacked onion or celery, finely diced apple, or seared wiener). Liberally stuff every pork cleave pocket with the blend. Season the two sides of the cleaves with Traeger Pork and Poultry Rub.

3) When prepared to cook, start the Traeger flame broil on Smoke with the cover open

until the fire is set up.

4) Arrange the hacks straightforwardly on the flame broil grind. Prepare for 45 to 50 minutes, or until the pork is cooked (160 degrees F on a moment read meat thermometer). There is no compelling reason to turn the cleaves. Allow the pork to rest for 2 to 3 minutes prior to moving to a platter or plates.

Pork Tenderloin:

Lean pork tenderloin can be scandalously dry—however not when covered with a flavourful combination. Utilize new spices on the off chance that you have them. Go with the pork with simmered or pureed potatoes and a green vegetable.

Ingredients:

1) 1/4 cup coarse-grain or Dijon-style mustard
2) 2 tablespoons honey
3) 2 tablespoons mayonnaise, for example, Hellmann's tablespoon cleaved

Method:

1) In a little bowl, join the mustard, honey, mayonnaise, parsley, and Traeger Pork and Poultry Rub; mix to blend. Lay the pork tenderloins in a level preparing dish. Pour the mustard-honey blend over the tenderloins, going to cover all sides. (If not cooking quickly, cover with cling wrap and refrigerate.)

2) When prepared to cook, start the Traeger barbecue on Smoke with the cover open until the fire is set up.

3) Lift the tenderloins out of the mustard-honey combination and orchestrate on an inclining on the flame broil grind. (Dispose of the excess mustard-honey blend.) 160 degrees F on a moment read meat thermometer. Cut into 3/4-inch cuts and serve.

Boneless Pork Ribs:

Nation style pork ribs come from the rib end of the sirloin and are extremely substantial, here and there weighing almost a half-pound each. Organic product-based grill sauces pair delightfully with them.

Ingredients:

1) 8 boneless nation style pork ribs
2) Traeger Pork and Poultry Rub, or your #1 grill rub
3) 1 Cup Traeger Apricot Barbecue Sauce, or your #1 natural product-based grill sauce

Method:

1) Start the Traeger flame broil on Smoke with the cover open until the fire is set up (4 to 5 minutes).

2) Arrange the pork ribs straightforwardly on the flame broil mesh and smoke for 60 minutes. Increment the temperature to 250 degrees F. Keep cooking for 1-1/2 hour to 2 hours, or until the ribs are delicate and have arrived at 155 degrees F on a moment read meat thermometer. Utilizing a seasoning brush, apply the Traeger Apricot Barbecue Sauce to the ribs, turning with utensils to arrive at all sides. Allow the ribs to rest for 3 minutes prior to serving.

Pulled Pork:

Pulled pork is a venture for a languid day. You can't surge it. The pork shoulder will take around 1-1/2 to 2 hours for every pound to cook flawlessly (190 degrees F), so start it promptly in the day in the event that you need to serve it for supper. A puckery vinegar-based sauce replaces grill sauce in Eastern North Carolina, where pulled pork is a religion. To make a Carolina-motivated sauce, join 2 cups of vinegar (white, apple juice, or a blend of both) with 1 tablespoon every one of earthy coloured sugar, salt, dark pepper, and hot sauce in a canning container. Add 2 teaspoons of squashed red pepper and let it sit for a few hours prior to serving. This stuff is hot, yet plays off the wealth of the pork.

Ingredients:

1) 1 bone-in pork shoulder broil (likewise called Boston butt), around 5 pounds, outside fat managed to around 1/8-INCh
2) Traeger Pork and Poultry Rub
3) 2 Cups squeezed apple in a food-safe shower bottle (discretionary)
4) Traeger Regular Barbecue Sauce
5) 10 cheeseburger buns

Method:

1) When prepared to cook, start the Traeger flame broil on Smoke with the top open until the fire is set up.

2) Put the meal on the flame broil grind, fat-side up, and cook for 3 hours, showering with squeezed apple consistently after the primary hour, whenever wanted. Move to an expendable aluminum foil container adequately huge to hold the meat, and meal for 5 or 6 extra hours, or until a moment read meat thermometer embedded in the thickest part, however not contacting bone, registers 190 degrees F. In the event that the pork begins to brown excessively, cover it freely with aluminum foil.

3) Allow it to rest for 30 minutes. On the other hand, you can wrap it firmly in foil and "hold" it in a protected cooler for as long as 60 minutes. Pour the juices from the lower part of the aluminium foil skillet into a sauce separator.

4) While the pork is as yet hot, manoeuvre it into lumps utilizing forks or your hands (ideally shielded from the warmth with lined, hard core elastic gloves). Dispose of the bone and any pieces of fat or connective tissue. Manoeuvre each lump into shreds, and move to a huge blending bowl. Season with extra rub, whenever wanted, and soak with the saved drippings (dispose of any fat that has

drifted to the highest point of the drippings). Add grill sauce, whenever wanted, and blend well. Or on the other hand serve the grill sauce as an afterthought.

Baked Ham:

Completely cooked hams, for example, the one called for in this formula, don't need to be warmed to 160 degrees F like a crude item. Indeed, you can serve them cold.

Ingredients:

1) 1 Whole bone-in ham
2) 1/4 cup arranged horseradish, or more to taste
3) 2 tablespoons Dijon-style mustard

Method:

1) If the ham actually has a layer of fat and skin on it, trim the skin off, leaving around 1/4-INCh of fat on the meat. Line a huge broiling skillet with aluminum foil, permitting it to overhang the sides. (This will make tidy up simpler.) Put the ham in the roaster.

2) In a pot, join the Traeger Apricot Barbecue Sauce, the horseradish, and the mustard. Warm tenderly when the ham is almost done.

3) When prepared to cook, start the Traeger flame broil on Smoke with the top open until

the fire is set up.

4) Barbecue grind and prepare for 2-1/2 hours, or until the inward temperature of the ham is 135 degrees F when perused on a moment read meat thermometer. Brush the apricot-horseradish coat over the outside of the ham. Keep on preparing for an hour more. Permit it to rest for 20 minutes prior to cutting and presenting with the excess apricot-horseradish coat, ideally warmed on the flame broil or burner.

Cheddar-Pork Burgers:

Exhausted with conventional beef burgers? Ground pork, prepared with grill rub and grill sauce, is a pleasant change. Coleslaw makes a marvellous backup.

Ingredients:

1) 2 pounds ground pork, cold
2) 1 Cup ground cheddar
3) 2 tablespoons ground onion (discretionary)
4) 4 burger buns, for serving
5) Your most loved sauces (cut onions, pickles, tomatoes, and so on)

Method:

1) Put the pork, cheddar, onion, if utilizing, Traeger Regular Barbecue Sauce, and Traeger Pork and Poultry Rub in a blending blend the meat, cheddar, and flavors. Rewet your hands if fundamental. Structure the meat combination into 4 equivalent patties, and utilize your thumbs to frame a huge shallow sadness on one side of every patty. (This will shield the burgers from protruding in the center when flame broiled.)

2) When prepared to cook, start the Traeger flame broil on Smoke with the top open until the fire is set up (4 to 5 minutes).

3) Arrange the burgers, sorrow side down, on the barbecue mesh and smoke for 30 minutes. Increment the temperature to 300 degrees F. Barbecue the burgers until a moment read meat thermometer peruses 160 degrees F, around 45 minutes. Turn the burgers part of the way through the barbecuing time. Let rest for 2 to 3 minutes prior to serving to let the juices rearrange themselves. Serve on buns with extra Traeger Regular Barbecue Sauce as well as your #1 toppings.

Teriyaki pork and pineapple skewers:

Once in a while, pork sirloin is sold in markets previously cubed and joined by wooden sticks. Typically, it is named "city chicken," a name it got during the Great Depression when pork was more affordable than chicken.

Ingredients:

1) 1-pound pork sirloin shapes, each about
2) 1-inch by 1-INCh and 1/2-inch thick (18 pieces)
3) 2 to 3 cuts new pineapple, cored and cut into reduced down pieces
4) 1 Cup Traeger Carne Asada Marinade, or your #1 teriyaki marinade
5) 6 enormous scallions (green onions), managed, pale and light green parts cut into 1-INCh lengths
6) 6 6-to 8-inch wooden sticks

Method:

1) Thread a pork shape through the dainty side on a stick, trailed by a lump of pineapple and a bit of green onion; rehash the arrangement twice to finish a stick (three 3D squares of pork per stick). Rehash with the other five sticks. Move the sticks to a glass container or pie plate and pour the marinade over them, going to cover on all sides.

2) When prepared to cook, start the Traeger flame broil on Smoke with the cover open

until the fire is set up.

3) Drain the sticks, disposing of the marinade. Mastermind the sticks on the flame broil mesh and barbecue, turning once, for 10 minutes, or until the pork is cooked through. Move the sticks to a platter or plates and serve right away.

Brats in a Bath:

This is an ideal formula for closely following or a game day party at home as the imps will remain hot for quite a while in their "shower". Whenever wanted, you can smoke the whelps prior to completing them over higher warmth.

Ingredients:

1) 3 to 4 12-OUnce jars of brew (dull or light)
2) 2 huge onions, stripped and cut into rings
3) 2 tablespoons spread, in addition to extra for buttering the buns
4) 10 whelps, uncooked
5) 10 whelp or hoagie buns
6) Mustard for serving

Method:

1) Empty the brew into a pot. Add the onions and 2 tablespoons of margarine. Bring to a stew on the burner.

2) When prepared to cook, start the Traeger barbecue on Smoke with the cover open until the fire is set up.

3) Put a profound dispensable aluminum foil skillet on one side of the Traeger. Cautiously pour the brew and onions from the pot into the skillet on the barbecue. Orchestrate the rascals on the opposite side of the flame broil grind. Flame broil the imps until cooked through, turning often with utensils, around 20 to 25 minutes. Move the rascals to the lager shower and cover the container firmly with aluminum foil. Let the whelps stew in the shower until the onions are delicate, 45 minutes to 60 minutes.

4) To serve, lift a rascal out of the shower and put it on a bun. Top it with onions and mustard, whenever wanted. This is an ideal formula for closely following or a game day party at home as the imps will remain hot for quite a while in their "shower". Whenever wanted, you can smoke the whelps prior to completing them over higher warmth.

Italian Milk-Braised Pork Tenderloin:

While pork braised in milk is notable in Italy, it is more uncommon here. It is a straightforward however delectable arrangement; the pork braises gradually in milk injected with new slashed rosemary and sage (utilize dried spices on the off chance that you should) and garlic. Try not to be concerned if the milk coagulates to some degree: It should. Simply separate the curds with a little speed as coordinated underneath

Ingredients:

1) 2 pork tenderloins, each around 1 pound
2) 2 tablespoons extra-virgin olive oil (partitioned use)
3) 2 tablespoons cleaved new rosemary, or 2 teaspoons dried
4) 2 tablespoons slashed new wise, or 2 teaspoons dried
5) Salt and newly ground dark pepper
6) 2 Cups entire milk, or cream
7) 1-1/2 teaspoons Worcestershire sauce
8) 2 Cloves garlic, crushed
9) 1 cove leaf

Method:

1) Trim the pork tenderloins of any additional fat or silver skin. Season the tenderloins with salt and pepper.

2) On the burner, heat an ovenproof skillet over medium-high warmth. Add the leftover tablespoon of olive oil to the skillet. Add the tenderloins and earthy colored well on all sides, turning with utensils.

3) When prepared to cook, start the Traeger flame broil on Smoke with the top open until the fire is set up.

4) Carefully move the skillet with the pork and milk to the flame broil grind. (In the event that you don't possess an ovenproof skillet, basically move the pork and milk combination to a heating dish and put that on the barbecue grind.) Braise for 60 minutes, or until the pork is delicate and the milk has incompletely vanished. (The inside temperature of the pork should be 160 degrees F.) Slice the pork into emblems and orchestrate on a platter. Eliminate the garlic cloves and sound leaf from the milk blend and dispose of. Whisk, at that point taste for preparing, adding more salt and pepper whenever wanted.

CHAPTER 4
Traeger Poultry

Poultry Tips:

1) Chicken should consistently be cooked to an inside temperature of 165 degrees F to slaughter food-borne microorganisms like salmonella.

2) Wash anything that has interacted with crude poultry altogether with hot foamy water (hands, cutting sheets, blades, platters, and so forth) prior to reusing.

3) Lightly smoke stripped, hard-cooked eggs on the Traeger for an intriguing turn on deviled eggs or egg serving of mixed greens. (Smoke for around 30 minutes. Longer, and the outside of the egg layer will harden.)

4) Whole chickens are generally more affordable than chicken parts. Figure out how to separate entire winged animals to set aside cash.

5) Brine poultry prior to cooking for additional sogginess and flavor. Blend 1/4 cup salt and 2 tablespoons of sugar with a quart of cold water; mix until the salt and sugar precious

stones disintegrate. Lower the poultry, at that point cover what's more, refrigerate. Saline solution entire chickens or turkeys short-term; salt water bosoms, thighs, and legs for 2 to 4 hours. Wash, at that point dry altogether prior to continuing with the formula.

6) Put aromatics, for example, onions, carrots, celery, spices, or cut-up lemons or oranges in the hole of a broiling feathered creature for additional flavor.

7) For better sautéing, rub the outside of the fowl with liquefied margarine or olive or vegetable oil prior to preparing.

8) Mix dried spices or slashed new spices and flavors into mollified spread, at that point refrigerate or freeze. Fold it under the skin of broiling chickens to add extravagance, clamminess, and flavor.

Basic Traeger Chicken Breast:

Boneless, skinless chicken bosoms aren't anything if not flexible. On a couple of moments' notifications, you can fix a fine feast for organization or family. You will be astonished by how sodden the bosoms are when flame broiled on a Traeger. Make additional items to have close by for servings of mixed greens, fajitas, nachos, sandwiches, and so on

Ingredients:

1) 8 boneless, skinless chicken bosoms, each around 6 ounces after tenders are taken out (see Note beneath)

Method:

1) When prepared to cook, start the Traeger flame broil on Smoke with the cover open until the fire is set up (4 to 5 minutes).

2) 8 boneless, skinless chicken bosoms, each around 6 ounces after tenders are eliminated (see Note underneath)

3) Arrange the chicken bosoms on the barbecue mesh and cook, turning once part of the way inside temperature, when perused on a moment read meat thermometer, is 170 degrees F.

4) Note: The little fold of meat on the underside of a chicken bosom is known as the delicate. Customarily, the butcher has just taken out it. The bosom will flame broil all the more uniformly and look more alluring on the off chance that you eliminate the delicate and barbecue it independently.

Brined chicken breasts with mandarin glaze:

Maybe you've known about "tenderizing," however have never attempted it. In its least difficult structure, tenderizing methods absorbing food pungent water for 30 minutes to a few hours. It has a perceptible effect in flavour, surface, and succulence particularly in poultry. This specific dish is extraordinary when presented with white rice.

Ingredients:

1) 2 quarts cold water
2) 1/2 Cup genuine salt, or 1/4 cup if utilizing table salt
3) 1/4 cup earthy colored sugar
4) 1/2 Cup soy sauce
5) 8 boneless, skinless chicken bosoms, each around 6 ounces after tenders are taken out (see Note beneath)
6) Traeger Mandarin Glaze, or Chinese sweet bean stew sauce or prepared sauce
7) 2 Scallions (green onions), managed and meagerly cut, for decorate (discretionary) Cause the saline solution: To pour into an enormous blending bowl and mix until the sugar and salt break up.
8) Lower the chicken bosoms in the saline solution, cover, and refrigerate for 2 to 4 hours (no more, if you don't mind Channel the

chicken and wipe off

Method:

1) When prepared to cook, start the Traeger barbecue on Smoke with the cover open until the fire is set up.

2) Arrange the chicken bosoms on the barbecue mesh and cook, turning once partially inside temperature, when perused on a moment read meat thermometer is 170 degrees F. Brush the chicken bosoms with the Traeger Mandarin Glaze during the most recent couple of minutes of cooking. Eliminate to a platter or plates and sprinkle the onions over the chicken bosoms, whenever wanted.

3) Note: The little fold of meat on the underside of a chicken bosom is known as the delicate. Regularly, the butcher has just eliminated it. The bosom will flame broil all the more uniformly and look more alluring in the event that you eliminate the delicate and barbecue it independently.

Barbecued Chicken Thighs:

Thighs are not just perhaps the most delicious piece of the chicken, yet they are frequently a deal at the meat counter. A short plunge in farm style dressing guarantees they'll be damp when you carry them to the table. Don't hesitate to substitute another dressing—Italian, Caesar, or vinaigrette—if that is the thing that you have in your wash room.

Ingredients:

1) Traeger Chicken Rub, or your number one poultry rub
2) 1 Cup farm style dressing
3) 1/2 teaspoon coarsely ground dark pepper

Method:

1) Trim the chicken thighs of any abundance fat. Season with the Traeger Chicken Rub.

2) In a huge blending bowl, consolidate the farm dressing and pepper, and mix to join. Add the chicken thighs and throw delicately with your hands to cover the thighs altogether. Whenever wanted, or cook right away.

3) When prepared to cook, start the Traeger flame broil on Smoke with the cover open until the fire is set up.

4) Lift the chicken from the marinade (dispose of any left in the bowl). Organize the chicken

thighs, skin-side down, on the flame broil grind. Flame broil for 40 to 45 minutes, or until the chicken arrives at 170 degrees F on a moment read meat thermometer. Try not to turn the chicken while it is cooking. Move the chicken to a platter or plates. Let rest for 2 minutes prior to serving.

5) Note: If you favor boneless skinless chicken thighs, abbreviate the cooking time to 30 minutes.

No Fuss Roasted Chicken:

Nothing muddled here. Simply oil the flying creature, season it, and let your Traeger do something amazing. In under 90 minutes, you'll have fresh skin and delicious meat with a trace of wood smoke. Complete two chickens, and you'll have extras to anticipate.

Ingredients:

1) One chicken, 4 to 5 pounds
2) Extra-virgin olive oil or vegetable oil
3) Traeger Chicken Rub, your number one rub, or salt and pepper

Method:

1) Wash the chicken all around with cold running water. Dry altogether with paper towels.

2) Oil the outside of the fledgling and season with the Traeger Chicken Rub. Fold the chicken wings behind the back. Tie the legs along with butcher's string. (This gives you a moister fowl and a more alluring introduction.)

3) When prepared to cook, start the Traeger barbecue on Smoke with the cover open until the fire is set up.

4) Place the chicken on the barbecue grind, bosom side up, and close the cover. Cook the chicken until a moment read meat thermometer embedded into the thickest piece of a thigh enrolls a temperature of 165 degrees F, 70 to an hour and a half. Eliminate the chicken to a platter and permit it to rest for 5 minutes. Unfasten the legs and cut.

Greek-Style Chicken with Garlic and Lemon:

Little potatoes threw in olive oil and salt and pepper and afterward broiled close by the chicken make a simple and flavourful side dish. A green plate of mixed greens balances the feast.

Ingredients:

1) 2 broiling chickens (3-1/2 to 4 pounds each), each cut into 8 pieces
2) 2 lemons, slice into quarters through the stem closes
3) 1 Cup chicken stock

Method:

1) Arrange the chicken pieces in a solitary layer in an enormous broiling skillet (whenever wanted, utilize an expendable aluminum foil simmering container). Press the juice from each bit of lemon over the chicken, getting any seeds in your fingers. Wrap the lemon skins up with the chicken. Sprinkle the olive oil over all.

2) Sprinkle the garlic over the chicken. Residue the chicken with the dried oregano, and season it liberally with one of the two recommended Traeger rubs, or salt and dark pepper. Empty the chicken stock into the container.

3) When prepared to cook, start the Traeger flame broil on Smoke with the top open until the fire is set up.

4) Move to a platter or plates and spoon a portion of the juices on top. Let rest for 3 minutes prior to serving.

Barbecued Chicken quarters:

Let's be honest: The grilled chicken of our childhood frequently guaranteed more than it conveyed. Scorched outwardly and crude within, it tried the guts of the most committed barbecue bosses of the day. With all due respect, they were by and large working with barbecues that were simply shallow container with a flame broil grind, barbecues that were intended for direct barbecuing as it were. Flare-ups were a rocking' roller. Not so with a Traeger, which barbecues by implication. Your chicken need not dread the fire.

Ingredients:

1) 6 leg and thigh quarters, around 5 to 6 pounds
2) Vegetable oil or extra-virgin olive oil
3) Traeger Chicken Rub, or your number one generally useful grill rub
4) 2 Cups Traeger Regular Barbecue Sauce, or your number one grill sauce

Method:

1) Wash the chicken under virus running water

2) Oil each quarter, at that point season with Traeger Chicken Rub.

3) When prepared to cook, start the Traeger flame broil on Smoke with the cover open until the fire is set up.

4) Arrange the chicken quarters on the flame broil grind, skin-side up. Broil for 1 to 1-1/2 hours, or until the inner temperature (embed the test of a moment read meat thermometer into the thickest piece of the thigh, however not contacting bone) peruses 165 degrees F. Utilizing a treating brush, apply grill sauce to the two sides of the chicken the most recent 15 minutes of cooking, turning once. (In the event that you apply the sauce too soon, the sugars in the sauce could caramelize and singe.)

Buffalo Chicken Wraps:

All the kinds of that American work of art—Buffalo wings—without the bones and in a simple to-eat structure! Chicken fingers are frequently a deal at the general store.

Ingredients:

1) 1-1/4 pounds chicken fingers
2) 3 tablespoons margarine
3) 1/2 Cup hot sauce, for example, Frank's Red-hot
4) 1-1/2 Cups destroyed lettuce
5) 1 Cup diced celery
6) 1/2 Cup arranged blue cheddar or farm dressing
7) 10-INCh flour tortillas

Method:

1) Season the chicken strips on all sides with the Traeger Cajun Shake or Pork and Poultry Shake.

2) When prepared to cook, start the Traeger barbecue on Smoke with the cover open until the fire is set up.

3) Arrange the chicken strips on the flame broil grind. While the chicken is cooking, liquefy the margarine in a pan. Add the hot sauce and mix to consolidate. Utilizing utensils, move the cooked chicken strips to the hot sauce blend, going to cover.

4) If wanted, quickly warm the tortillas on the flame broil. (They are simpler to deal with when warm.) Lay the tortillas on a level work surface. Utilizing utensils, lift the chicken strips from the sauce and orchestrate on the tortillas. Top with the lettuce and celery.

Shower with the blue cheddar or farm dressing, and move up, burrito-style. Serve right away.

Basic Beer Can Chicken:

Brew can chicken is currently a staple in North American lawns. Furthermore, in light of current circumstances: it's super-clammy. In any case, truly, you don't need to utilize brew. Canned organic product juice, tea, soft drink, and so forth, work similarly also. Ensure your model of Traeger barbecue has enough leeway to oblige your upstanding chicken prior to beginning this formula. Supplant the lager jars with 6-ounce natural product or vegetable juice jars. Cooking time will be marginally less—around one hour all out.

Ingredients:

1) 1 3-1/2-to-4-pound chicken, giblets eliminated
2) 1 12-OUnce container of brew

Method:

1) Eliminate any additional fat from the body and neck pits. Wash the chicken, inside Hickory, Alder, Oak, Pecan also, out, with cold running water. Channel and smear dry with paper towels. Move the chicken to a preparing skillet. Overlay the wing tips despite the chicken's good faith.

2) Open the brew and empty half into a glass. (How you manage the brew in the glass is up to you.) Using a "congregation key" can opener, make an extra opening or two in the top of the lager can. Set it in the heating skillet. This shields the rub from going all over the place and makes it simpler to ship to the barbecue. Cautiously facilitate the chicken onto the brew can so they can rest in the body cavity. Bring the legs of the chicken forward so they structure a mount with the lager can. Final detail any spots where the rub was upset.

3) When prepared to cook, start the Traeger flame broil on Smoke with the cover open until the fire is set up.

4) Carefully move the chicken on its brew can to the flame broil grind, situating it where the barbecue cover is most noteworthy. Cook the chicken until the skin is brilliant earthy colored and the inside temperature embedded in the thickest piece of the thigh peruses 170 degrees F on a moment read meat thermometer, around 1-1/4 to /2 hours. In the event that the highest point of the chicken browns excessively fast, cover it freely with aluminum foil. Cautiously move the chicken on its can to a platter or clean heating container. Cut and serve.

Cheesy Chicken Enchiladas:

This dish is a genuine group pleaser, yet possibly takes minutes to gather on the off chance that you have the cooked chicken close by from a past Traeger barbecue meeting. (Cooked turkey can sub for the chicken.) Serve with rice, refried dark beans, and destroyed lettuce and radishes.

Ingredients:

1) 6 cups destroyed or cubed cooked chicken
2) 3 cups ground Mexican-mix cheddar, or Monterey Jack or gentle Cheddar (12 ounces), partitioned use
3) 1 Cup acrid cream or Mexican crema
4) 1 Cup pitted cut dark olives
5) 1 4-ounce can cleave green chiles
6) 2 10-OUnce jars green or red enchilada sauce (separated use)
7) 12 8-inch flour tortillas
8) 3 scallions (green onions), managed, white and green parts daintily cut, for serving (discretionary)
9) Fresh cilantro leaves, hacked, for serving (discretionary)

Method:

1) Make the filling: In a huge blending bowl, join the cooked chicken and 2 Cups of the cheddar. Mix in the acrid cream, dark olives, and green chiles and blend well.

2) Pour one container of the enchilada sauce into the lower part of a 13-by 9-inch preparing dish. Spoon around 1/3 cup of the filling on the lower third of every tortilla and move up. Move to the preparing dish, long sides of the enchiladas contacting. At the point when you have gathered the entirety of the tortillas, pour the second container of enchilada sauce over the tops, utilizing a spoon or spatula to cover the outside of every tortilla with the sauce. Sprinkle the leftover cup of cheddar down the focal point of the column of moved tortillas. Cover the preparing dish firmly with foil.

3) When prepared to cook, start the Traeger barbecue on Smoke with the cover open until the fire is set up.

4) Bake the enchiladas for 30 minutes. At that point eliminate the foil, and heat for 15 additional minutes, or until the enchiladas are hot and the cheddar is softened. Enhancement with cut scallions and hacked new cilantro, whenever wanted. Serve hot.

First Timer's Turkey:

When you have Traeger in your group. It couldn't be simpler. Sauce making by enlisting a capable sauce moister or purchasing a decent quality jolted sauce. While numerous individuals cut the turkey bosom with their blade corresponding to the bosom bone, we've thought that it was' smarter to eliminate the whole bosom and afterward cut it across. That way, every individual who loves white meat gets both meat and skin.

Ingredients:

1) 1 turkey (defrosted if recently frozen)
2) You'll additionally require: an enormous strong simmering container; butcher's string; a moment read meat thermometer

Method:

1) (In the event that your turkey accompanied a sauce parcel, eliminate that, as well.) Wash the turkey all around with cold running water and wipe off with paper towels. Investigate the winged animal for any leftover quills, and eliminate these with kitchen tweezers.

2) Position the turkey in the broiling skillet and brush it equitably On the off chance that your turkey accompanied a string sling for simple expulsion from the dish once the fledgling is simmered, position it under the winged animal as per the bundle headings.

3) When prepared to cook, start the Traeger flame broil on Smoke with the top open until the fire is set up.

4) Put the broiling dish with the turkey straightforwardly on the barbecue grind. Cook the turkey for 3 hours. Addition the test from the meat thermometer in the thickest piece of the thigh, however not contacting bone: You're searching for a temperature of 165 degrees F. The turkey ought to likewise be flawlessly sautéed with fresh skin. In the event that the temperature is not as much as that, or if your turkey isn't seared as you would prefer, let it cook for an additional 30 minutes, at that point check the temperature once more. Rehash until the turkey is completely cooked.

5) When the turkey is done, cautiously move it to a cutting board and let it rest for 20 minutes. Try not to tent it with aluminum foil or the skin will lose its freshness.

6) Carve and serve.

Smoked Turkey Legs:

Event congregations and fairs have given smoked turkey legs a faction like after, with certain individuals offering cash online for a formula that copies the legs sold at Disneyland. The mystery is to absorb the legs salt water for 24 hours, at that point smoke them low and moderate. The flavour is ham-like, and addictive.

Ingredients:

1) 1-gallon cold water
2) 1 Cup Morton's Tender Quick
3) 1/4 cup earthy colored sugar
4) 6 allspice berries, squashed (discretionary)
5) 6 entire dark peppercorns
6) 2 inlet leaves, broken into pieces
7) 6 entire cloves

Method:

1) In a huge stockpot, consolidate one gallon of water, the rub, relieving salt, earthy colored sugar, allspice (if utilizing), peppercorns, inlet leaves, cloves, and fluid smoke. Cool to room temperature, at that point refrigerate until completely chilled. Add the turkey legs, ensuring they're totally lowered in the saline solution.

2) After 24 hours, channel the turkey legs and dispose of the salt water. Flush the saline solution off the legs with cold water, at that point dry altogether with paper towels. Get over any sticking strong flavors.

3) When prepared to cook, start the Traeger flame broil on Smoke with the cover open until the fire is set up.

4) Lay the turkey legs straightforwardly on the barbecue grind. (Ensure the test doesn't contact bone or you'll get a bogus perusing.) The turkey legs should be profoundly seared. Try not to be frightened if the meat under the skin is pinkish: That's a substance response to the fix and the smoke called a "smoke ring". Serve quickly, or refrigerate.

5) Note: If you can't discover these Flintstone-sequel legs, you can substitute more modest ones. Lessen the cooking time likewise.

CHAPTER 5

Traeger Lamb

Lamb Tips:

1) Lamb edge or round-bone shoulder cleaves are frequently altogether more affordable than rib or flank slashes.

2) Buy grass-took care of sheep when feasible for the best surface and flavor.

3) Marinate sheep short-term in packaged vinaigrette or a marinade making.

4) Lamb shanks are astounding when cooked low and delayed on your Traeger in an appetizing fluid. (Cover firmly and permit at any rate four hours for the shanks to get delicate.)

5) Butterflied boneless leg of sheep is a brisk and simple supper for a weeknight. Generally, it is rolled and made sure about with flexible netting. Essentially eliminate the netting prior to marinating or preparing the sheep, at that point lay level on the barbecue grind.

6) The wealth of sheep can be offset with acids,

for example, wine, vinegar, or lemon juice.

Rack of Lamb:

Numerous plans for rack of sheep call for it to be burned in hot oil prior to simmering. Yet, there's no need: The prepared sheep can go directly into the Traeger. The expression "frenched" alludes to a slash—normally sheep or veal—that has had the rib bones scratched for a more alluring introduction on the plate.

Ingredients:

1) 1 8-bone rack of sheep, 1-1/2 pounds, frenched and cut back of abundance excess
2) 2 tablespoons new spices, for example, rosemary, parsley, or thyme, or two teaspoons dried

Method:

1) Rub the rack of sheep with olive oil and season with Traeger Prime Rib Rub and the spices.

2) When prepared to cook, start the Traeger barbecue on Smoke with the top open until the fire is set up top shut, for 10 to 15 minutes.

3) Place the sheep on the barbecue grind, gathered side together. Cook for 30 minutes

for medium uncommon (135 degrees F on a moment read meat thermometer embedded into the focal point of the meat, yet not contacting bone), longer in the event that you like your sheep less uncommon.

4) Transfer the sheep to a cutting board and let it rest for 5 minutes. Cut into 2-BONE areas.

Roast Leg of Lamb:

Butterflied boneless leg of sheep is frequently sold folded into a dish like shape and held along with mesh. You can leave it in the netting whenever wanted, however a moved meal for every pound, or until it arrives at medium-uncommon. You can cook bone-in sheep a similar way. The marinade beneath is additionally phenomenal on rack of sheep and sheep cleaves.

Ingredients:

1) One lemon, washed
2) 1/4 cup red wine vinegar
3) 4 cloves garlic, minced
4) 2 tablespoons minced new rosemary leaves, or 2 teaspoons dried
5) 2 teaspoons new thyme, minced, or 1 teaspoon dried
6) 1 teaspoon salt
7) 1 teaspoon newly ground dark pepper
8) 1 Cup extra-virgin olive oil

9) 1 onion, cut into rings
10) 1 4-to 5-pound butterflied (boneless) leg of sheep

Method:

1) Crush Walnut, Cherry, Apple the juice into a blending bowl, saving the lemon skins. Speed in the olive oil. Eliminate any netting from the sheep. Put the sheep into an enormous resealable plastic sack. Back rub the pack to convey the marinade and spices. Refrigerate for a few hours, or overnight.

2) Remove the sheep from the marinade and wipe off with paper towels. Dispose of the marinade.

3) When prepared to cook, start the Traeger barbecue on Smoke with the cover open until the fire is set up.

4) Arrange the sheep on the flame broil grind, fat-side down. Flame broil 10 to 15 minutes for every side for medium-uncommon (135 degrees F on a moment read meat thermometer), longer in the event that you favor your sheep all the more very much done. Let rest for 5 minutes. Cut daintily across the grain, and serve.

Grilled Lamb Chops with Chili-Mint Sauce:

Little, delicious sheep slashes are extraordinary possibility for "Trailering." They are best when served medium-uncommon.

Ingredients:

1) 8 flank sheep slashes, 3/4-inch thick (around 4 to 5 ounces each), or sheep rib cleaves
2) 1/2 Cup refined white vinegar or white wine
3) 1 teaspoon salt
4) 1/2 teaspoon newly ground dark pepper
5) 2 tablespoons ground or finely minced onion
6) 1 tablespoon new mint, slashed
7) 2 tablespoons extra-virgin olive oil
8) 1/2 Cup mint jam

Method:

1) Using a sharp blade, cut back any overabundance excess off the sheep cleaves and move the slashes to a huge resealable plastic sack. In a little blending bowl, join the vinegar and salt and pepper and mix until the salt disintegrates. Mix in the onion, mint, and olive oil. Pour over the sheep slashes and refrigerate for 2 to 4 hours.

2) Drain the sheep slashes and wipe off with paper towels. Season on the two sides with the Traeger Prime Rib Rub, or salt and pepper.

3) When prepared to cook, start the Traeger flame broil on Smoke with the cover open until the fire is set up.

4) Arrange the hacks on the flame broil grind. Flame broil for 4 to 6 minutes for each side for medium-uncommon (130 to 135 degrees F on a moment read meat thermometer). In the interim, consolidate the mint jam and the Traeger Mandarin Glaze Sauce in a little pot. Warm on the burner or flame broil until the jam is dissolved, blending sporadically. Present with the sheep hacks.

CHAPTER 6
Traeger Seafood

Glazed Salmon:

A cafe type feast in around 30 minutes? It's conceivable with your Traeger. Particularly in the event that you approach new wild-got salmon, ideally from the Pacific. Lemon wedges and twigs of new tarragon or dill will give your plates visual allure.

Ingredients:

1) 4 focus cut salmon filets with skin on, every 6 to 8-ounces
2) Traeger Salmon Shake, or salt and newly ground dark pepper
3) 1/2 Cup mayonnaise, ideally Hellmann's
4) 2 tablespoons Dijon-style mustard
5) 1 tablespoon new lemon juice
6) 1 tablespoon slashed new tarragon or dill, or 1 teaspoon dried

Method:

1) Season the filets with the Traeger Salmon Shake. Make the coating: Combine the mayonnaise and mustard in a little bowl. Mix

in the lemon juice and tarragon. Spread the substance side of the filets with the coating.

2) When prepared to cook, start the Traeger barbecue on Smoke with the top open until the fire is set up.
3) Arrange the salmon filets on the barbecue grind, skin-side down. Flame broil for 25 to 30 minutes, or until the salmon is dark and pieces effectively with a fork. Move to a platter or plates and serve right away.

Cedar-Planked Salmon:

While this is a noteworthy supper for organization, it is simple enough for a bustling weeknight dinner. Any extra Lemon-Dill Butter combines delightfully with flame broiled shrimp.

Ingredients:

1) 1 lemon
2) 8 tablespoons (1 stick) margarine, at room temperature
3) 2 tablespoons new dill, hacked
4) Traeger Salmon Shake, or salt and newly ground dark pepper
5) 4 skinless salmon filets, ideally focus cut (6-to 8-ounces each)
6) 1 untreated cedar board (around 16-by 8-inches), absorbed water to cover for 60 minutes, at that point depleted

Method:

1) Wash the lemon, and cut it down the middle through its equator. Cut one-half into slight cuts with a sharp blade and hold (dispose of stem end).

2) Eliminate the yellow zing from the other half with a blade or vegetable peeler and finely mince, or utilize a zester. Press the juice from the zested half, disposing of any seeds.

3) Make the Lemon-Dill Butter: In a little blending bowl, join the margarine with the lemon zing, 1 tablespoon of lemon squeeze, the dill, and 1-1/2 teaspoons Traeger Salmon Shake or 1 teaspoon of salt and 1/2 teaspoon newly ground dark pepper. Put in a safe spot or cover and refrigerate if not utilizing right away. (The Lemon-Dill Butter can likewise be frozen for as long as a half year.)

4) When prepared to cook, start the Traeger flame broil on Smoke with the top open until the fire is set up (4 to 5 minutes). Put the cedar board straightforwardly on the barbecue grind. (This is a more extended preheat than expected on the grounds that you need to get the board hot.)

5) Remove any pin bones from the salmon filets (you can feel the bones with your fingertips) with kitchen tweezers or needle-nosed forceps. Season the salmon filets on the two sides with Traeger Salmon Shake. Mastermind the filets on the board, and top each filet with a cut of lemon. Cook, top shut, for 25 to 30 minutes, or until the salmon is obscure and

pieces effectively when squeezed with a fork. Top each filet with a pat of Lemon-Dill Butter. Cautiously move the filets to a platter or plates and serve right away.

6) Note: A rimmed cookie sheet functions admirably for splashing the board. Keep it lowered by resting something hefty, similar to a supper plate, on the board.

Baked Cod:

For a simple side dish, cut the tops off ready tomatoes. Salt and pepper them, at that point top them with ground Parmesan or Romano cheddar and residue with dried basil. Heat the tomatoes close by the fish.

Ingredients:

1) 4 pieces cod flank (each around 8-ounces)
2) Juice of 1 lemon
3) 1/2 Cup (1 Stick) margarine, dissolved (separated use)
4) Traeger Salmon Shake, or salt and newly ground dark pepper
5) 25 round rich nibble saltines, for example, Ritz, squashed into fine pieces
6) 1-1/2 teaspoons dried basil
7) Chopped new parsley for embellish

Method:

1) Arrange the cod in a buttered 9-by 13-inch heating dish and shower it with the lemon juice and 1/4 cup of the liquefied spread. Join the wafer pieces, the basil, and the rest of the margarine in a little bowl and mix to blend. Top the cod with the morsel combination.

2) When prepared to cook, start the Traeger flame broil on Smoke with the top open until the fire is set up.

3) Put the preparing dish on the barbecue grind and heat for 20 minutes, or until the garnish is brilliant earthy colored and the fish pieces effectively when squeezed with a fork. Topping with parsley, whenever wanted.

Scallops:

When purchasing new scallops, make certain to search for ones that are marked "dry pack". This implies they have not been treated with phosphates, a synthetic frequently used to safeguard them until they will advertise.

Ingredients:

1) 1-1/2 pounds "large" scallops (10 to 15 for each pound)
2) 6 tablespoons margarine

3) 1 Clove garlic, minced
4) 1 tablespoon new lemon juice
5) Traeger Salmon Shake, or salt and newly ground dark pepper
6) Chopped new parsley for serving (discretionary)
7) Lemon wedges for serving

Method:

1) Line a rimmed preparing sheet with aluminum foil. Flush the scallops under virus running water and delicately dry on paper towels. Move them to the preparing sheet.

2) In a pot, liquefy the spread. Add the garlic and lemon juice. Eliminate from the warmth. Brush the scallops on the two sides with the garlic spread, at that point season with the Traeger Salmon Shake.

3) When prepared to cook, start the Traeger barbecue on Smoke with the cover open until the fire is set up.

4) Remove the scallops from the heating sheet and orchestrate the scallops straightforwardly on the flame broil grind. Move the scallops to a platter or plates. Sprinkle with parsley, whenever wanted, and present with lemon wedges.

Texas Cowboy Shrimp:

Ingredients:

1) 2 pounds enormous shrimp, stripped and deveined (24 shrimp)
2) 3 tablespoons olive oil or vegetable oil
3) Salt and coarsely ground dark pepper
4) 1 Small onion, stripped and finely diced
5) 2 Cloves garlic, minced
6) 1/2 to 1 jalapeno pepper, cultivated and finely minced (discretionary)
7) Fresh cilantro leaves, cleaved

Method:

1) Wash the shrimp under virus running water, channel, and wipe off with paper towels. Move to a bowl. Delicately blend the shrimp in with 2 tablespoons of the oil, at that point season well with salt and pepper.
2) Heat a pot over medium-low warmth with 1 tablespoon of oil. Add the onion, garlic, and jalapeno pepper, whenever wanted, and sauté until mellowed. Mix in the grill sauce and keep warm.

3) When prepared to cook, start the Traeger flame broil on Smoke with the top open until the fire is set up.

4) Arrange the shrimp on the flame broil mesh and barbecue, 2 to 3 minutes for every side, until the shrimp is firm and dark and cooked through. Rapidly add the cooked shrimp to the warm sauce, alongside the cilantro. Mix tenderly to cover. Transform onto a platter or into a huge bowl and serve right away.

Citrus-Grilled Swordfish:

This is a simple method to plan firm, mellow tasting fish like monkfish, Chilean ocean bass, halibut, and so on

Method:

1) Slice the grapefruit into eighths. (In the event that utilizing the oranges and lime, cut each natural product into quarters.) Rub every swordfish steak on the two sides with olive oil. Season with Traeger Salmon Shake.

2) When prepared to cook, start the Traeger barbecue on Smoke with the top open until the fire is set up.

3) Arrange the swordfish steaks on the barbecue grind. Press the citrus juice (from 2 to 3

wedges of grapefruit) over the highest point of the steaks. Flame broil for 6 to 8 minutes. Utilizing a slender spatula, turn the steaks. Once more, crush citrus juice over the highest point of the steaks. Wrap up cooking the steaks, 6 to 8 minutes more, or until the substance is hazy and breaks into firm pieces when squeezed with a fork. Get done with a last press of citrus juice.

4) Note: Citrus organic products will yield more squeeze on the off chance that you microwave them for 20 to 30 seconds first.

Mediterranean Relish:

Storeroom things can be transformed into a scrumptious relish for swordfish or other firm-fleshed fish like fish, monkfish, salmon, or swordfish.

Ingredients:

1) 1/2 Cup pitted green olives, cleaved
2) 1/2 Cup pitted dark olives, cleaved
3) 1/4 cup sun-dried tomatoes, depleted of oil, and cleaved
4) 1/4 cup slashed onion
5) 1 Clove garlic, minced
6) 1 tablespoon red wine vinegar or newly crushed lemon juice
7) 3 tablespoons extra-virgin olive oil, in addition to additional for brushing the fish
8) Coarse salt and newly ground dark pepper
9) 4 6-ounce halibut steaks, each around 3/4-inch

thick, or another firm-fleshed fish

Method:

1) Make the relish: In a little blending bowl, join the green and dark.
2) When prepared to cook, start the Traeger barbecue on Smoke with the cover open until the fire is set up.

3) Misty and chips effectively when squeezed with a fork. Move to a platter or plates and top every steak with the olive relish.

Peppered Tuna:

Fish, tomatoes, mozzarella, and olive oil summon the island of Sicily, simply under the sole of the Italian boot. Go with great dried-up bread.

Ingredients:

1) 4 fish steaks (around 1-INCh thick, 6 to 8 ounces each)
2) 1/2 Cup extra-virgin olive oil
3) Coarsely ground dark pepper
4) Coarse salt (fit or ocean)
5) Half quart (2 Cups) cherry tomatoes, washed and divided longwise
6) 4 ounces mozzarella, ideally new, cut into reduced down pieces
7) 6 leaves new basil, slashed, or 1 teaspoon, dried

8) Lemon wedges, for serving

Method:

1) Trim any skin or dull spots off the tuna, if important. Oil the two sides of every steak.

2) Liberally season with coarsely ground dark pepper and salt to taste. In a little bowl, join 1/2 teaspoon dark pepper and 1/2 teaspoon salt with the vinegar and mix until the salt breaks up. Rush in the excess olive oil, and mix in the basil. In a bigger bowl, consolidate the tomatoes and mozzarella. Put in a safe spot.

3) When prepared to cook, start the Traeger flame broil on Smoke with the top open until the fire is set up.

4) Arrange the fish steaks on the flame broil mesh and barbecue, turning once, until the steaks are seared outwardly and the ideal level of doneness is reached, 3 to 4 minutes for each side for uncommon—longer for fish that is completely cooked (roughly 8 to 10 minutes for every side). Rewhips the dressing, pour over the tomatoes and mozzarella, and throw delicately.

5) Move the fish steaks to plates and split the tomato and mozzarella serving of mixed greens between them. (Plate with the plate of mixed greens just to the side of the fish.) Serve with lemon wedges for crushing.

Lobster Tail:

A strong pair of kitchen shears—or even tin clips—will help you discharge the delicious lobster meat from the intense.The base of the tail is a famous method of introducing lobster in eateries.

Ingredients:

1) 8 tablespoons margarine
2) 2 tablespoons new lemon juice
3) 1 teaspoon paprika
4) 1/2 teaspoon garlic salt
5) 1/4 teaspoon newly ground dark pepper
6) 2 tablespoons new parsley, cleaved

Method:

1) Prepare the lobster by chopping down the center of the extreme shell toward the tail with kitchen shears. Utilizing your fingers, delicately pry the meat from the shell, keeping it appended at the base of the tail. Lift the meat so it is laying on top of the split shell. Spot the lobster tails on a rimmed preparing sheet.

2) Melt the spread in a little pan over medium-low warmth. Rush in the lemon juice, paprika, garlic salt, pepper, and parsley (if utilizing). Pour around 1 tablespoon of the margarine blend over every lobster tail. Keep the excess spread combination warm.

3) When prepared to cook, start the Traeger flame broil on Smoke with the cover open until the fire is set up.

4) Remove the lobster tails from the heating sheet and orchestrate them straightforwardly on the flame broil grind. Move the lobster tails to a platter or plates. Present with the held spread blend.

CHAPTER 7
Traeger Vegetables

Cauliflower Medley:

Ingredients:

1) 1 huge head broccoli, cut into scaled down florets
2) 1 enormous head cauliflower, cut into scaled down florets
3) Extra-virgin olive oil
4) Traeger Veggie Shake, or salt and newly ground dark pepper

Method:

1) Put the vegetables on a rimmed heating sheet in a solitary layer. Sprinkle olive oil over the vegetables, going them to cover. Season with Traeger Veggie Shake.

2) When prepared to cook, start the Traeger barbecue on Smoke with the top open until the fire is set up.

3) Arrange the heating sheet on the barbecue

grind. Barbecue the vegetables, turning more than once, for 25 to 30 minutes, or until they are delicate and marginally seared. Move to a bowl or plates and serve right away.

Grilled Vegetable Salad:

The gem like shades of this serving of mixed greens will make it a gem on your supper table. On the off chance that there are extras, cut them into scaled down pieces and throw with cooked pasta.

Ingredients:

1) 1 red chime pepper
2) 1 orange or yellow chime pepper
3) 4 zucchini squash, ideally of uniform size
4) 4 yellow squash, ideally of uniform size
5) 1 pack asparagus
6) Extra-virgin olive oil
7) Traeger Veggie Shake
8) 1 lemon, quartered and cultivated
9) 1/2 Cup ground Parmesan cheddar
10) 2 tablespoons hacked new spices, such as parsley, basil, or oregano

Method:

1) When prepared to cook, start the Traeger barbecue on Smoke with the top open until the fire is set up.

2) Lay the chime peppers on the flame broil

mesh and burn on all sides, turning varying with utensils, 15 to 20 minutes altogether. Let cool somewhat, at that point strip the slender skin off (don't stress on the off chance that you can't get it all). Eliminate the stem, ribs, and center from each, and cut into slight strips. Save.

3) Meanwhile, trim the finishes off the squash and cautiously cut longwise into 1/4-inch cuts. Lay on a rimmed heating sheet in one layer. Trim the intense finishes off the asparagus (in the event that you twist a tail, it will break where it's delicate). Lay it across the squash. Shower or brush olive oil on the vegetables.

4) Arrange the squash and asparagus straightforwardly on the flame broil grind. (Lay the asparagus opposite to the bars of the mesh so the stalks don't fail to work out.) Keep the heating sheet close by. Flame broil the squash cuts for 2 to 3 minutes for each side, or until they are delicate, turning with utensils. Flame broil the asparagus until delicate, prodding with utensils to turn, 8 to 10 minutes complete. As the vegetables are done, move them to the heating sheet.

5) Arrange the vegetables, including the held ringer pepper, alluringly on a huge platter. Shower with extra olive oil, at that point crush lemon juice over all. Sprinkle uniformly with the Parmesan and spices. Serve at room temperature.

Steakhouse-Style Baked Potatoes:

For a modest yet merry weeknight dinner, set up a "potato bar" with heated potatoes and any backups your family enjoys, from bacon pieces to cut cured jalapenos.

Ingredients:

1) 4 extra-huge preparing potatoes, for example, Idaho
2) Traeger Beef Rub, or coarse salt, (for example, fit or ocean) and coarsely ground dark pepper
3) Butter
4) Sour cream
5) Fresh chives or scallions (green onions), managed and meagerly cut

Method:

1) Scrub the outside of the potatoes completely under virus running water with a vegetable brush. Dry with paper towels. Rub the oil over every potato, season liberally with the Traeger Beef Rub, and enclose by aluminum foil.

2) When prepared to cook, start the Traeger barbecue on Smoke with the cover open until the fire is set up.

3) Arrange the potatoes straightforwardly on the barbecue grind and prepare until delicate, around 1 to 1-1/4 hours. (To test for doneness, run a stick or blade through the focal point of a potato: It should experience with no opposition.) Utilizing a sharp blade, cut a longwise cut in each to allow the steam to get away. Crush the limited finishes of the potato to "lighten" it up. Serve promptly with spread, acrid cream, and chives.

Bean Casserole:

We've seen adaptations that utilization natively constructed cream of mushroom soup and even French-seared shallots in lieu of the customary firm onion beating. Yet, there are a few things you just shouldn't play with.

Ingredients:

1) 2 16-OUnce jars green beans, depleted, or 1-1/2 pounds new green beans, managed and cooked until delicate
2) 1/2 Cup milk
3) 2 teaspoons soy sauce
4) 1/2 teaspoon Worcestershire sauce
5) 1/2 teaspoon newly ground dark pepper
6) 1-1/3 cups French-singed onions, partitioned use
7) 1/4 cup finely diced red ringer pepper or jolted pimentos

Method:

1) In a blending bowl, join the beans, soup, milk, soy sauce, Worcestershire sauce, dark utilizing. Move to a 1-1/2-quart goulash dish.

2) When prepared to cook, start the Traeger barbecue on Smoke with the cover open until the fire is set up.

3) Cook the goulash until the filling is hot and percolating, 35 to 40 minutes. Top with the excess onions and cook for 5 to 10 minutes more, or until the onions are fresh and starting to brown.

Mushroom "burgers":

Substantial tasting Portobello mushrooms, marinated, implanted with wood smoke, and finished off with barbecued onions and cheddar, won't just satisfy any veggie lovers at your table—the carnivores will be fulfilled, as well. Regardless of whether you practice "Meatless Mondays" or not, check these out.

Ingredients:

1) 4 enormous Portobello mushrooms, every 4-to 5-creeps
2) 1 onion, stripped and cut into 1/2-INCh adjusts
3) 4 ounces mozzarella or muenster cheddar, meagerly cut
4) 1 huge ready tomato, daintily cut
5) 4 tablespoons spread, dissolved
6) 4 huge Kaiser-style cheeseburger moves, split
7) 1 enormous ready tomato, meagerly cut

Method:

1) Wipe the mushroom covers clean with a clammy paper towel. Eliminate the stems. Put the mushrooms and the onion cuts into a resealable pack alongside Channel. You can refrigerate the marinade and reuse whenever wanted, since it just contacted vegetables, and not meat.

2) When prepared to cook, start the Traeger barbecue on Smoke with the cover open until the fire is set up (4 to 5 minutes).

3) Arrange the mushrooms (gill-side down) and onion cuts on the barbecue mesh and smoke for 30 minutes. Increment delicate. The onions can even now hold a touch of crunch. At the point when the mushrooms are nearly done, top each with one-fourth of the cheddar. Brush the cut sides of the moves with the dissolved

margarine. Barbecue, cut-side down, for a couple of moments, or until they simply start to brown.

4) Transfer the base parts of the buns to plates or a platter. Top with the cheddar filled mushroom, onion cuts, tomato, pickle, lettuce leaves, and bun tops.

Smoke-Roasted Onion, Bacon, And Tomato Salad:

This interesting serving of mixed greens is magnificent with flame broiled meats. You can do a large part of the planning early—broil the onions, cook the bacon, and make the vinaigrette.

Ingredients:

1) 1 half quart cherry tomatoes, divided
2) 1 English cucumber, meagerly cut
3) 2 Cups crunchy lettuce, (for example, ice shelf or Romaine), coarsely hacked
4) 1 Cup bread garnishes for serving, ideally natively constructed
5) 1/2 Cup coarsely ground Parmesan cheddar

Method:

1) When prepared to cook, start the Traeger barbecue on Smoke with the cover open until the fire is set up (4 to 5 minutes).

2) Arrange the onions on the barbecue grind. Smoke for 30 minutes. Wrap the onions exclusively in aluminum foil and re-visitation of the flame broil.

3) Cook the onions until they are delicate, around 1 hour more. At the point when they are adequately cool to deal with, eliminate and dispose of the foil. Coarsely hack the onions, disposing of the finishes.

4) Meanwhile, in an enormous blending bowl, consolidate the vinegar, salt, and pepper. Gradually speed in the oil. Add the bacon disintegrates, onion, tomato, cucumber, and lettuce. Delicately prepare the fixings (clean hands function admirably for this) until the plate of mixed greens is covered with the dressing. Move to an alluring serving of mixed greens bowl or profound platter. Top with the bread garnishes and the Parmesan.

Grilled corn with bacon butter:

Corn and bacon go really well together.

Ingredients:

1) 3 segments of bacon
2) 12 tablespoons margarine
3) 2 teaspoons apple juice vinegar
4) 1 teaspoon Worcestershire sauce
5) 8 ears new sweet corn in their husks

Method:

1) Make the bacon spread: Starting in a virus skillet, fry the bacon over medium warmth until it is cooked and fresh. Channel on paper towels. Mince finely. In a little blending bowl, consolidate the bacon, margarine, scallion, Traeger Veggie Shake, vinegar, and Worcestershire sauce. Blend altogether with a wooden spoon. If not utilizing quickly, cover and refrigerate. (The spread will save for at any rate seven days.)

2) Eliminate all the silk. Leave the husks joined, however pull off any silk sticking to them.

3) When prepared to cook, start the Traeger flame broil on Smoke with the top open until the fire is set up.

4) Arrange the ears of corn straightforwardly on the flame broil grind. Barbecue for 12 to 14 minutes, turning every now and again, until a

portion of the parts are brilliant earthy colored. (The corn will brown unevenly.) Serve quickly with the bacon spread.

Barbecued Pinto Beans:

For comfort, this formula utilizes canned pinto beans; evaporated ones take to six hours to cook to non-abrasiveness. Heavenly with brisket, ribs, fajitas, or grilled pork steak or shoulder.

Ingredients:

1) 3 cuts bacon, chilly, diced
2) 1 onion, stripped and diced
3) 1/2 green chime pepper, cultivated and diced
4) 2 Cloves garlic, minced
5) 1 Cup brew, ideally Mexican, in addition to more if necessary
6) 1/2 Cup fermented espresso
7) 2 tablespoons molasses
8) 2 tablespoons salted jalapeno, minced, or more to taste (discretionary)
9) 3 15-OUnce jars pinto beans

Method:

1) Put the diced bacon in a cool skillet. Turn the warmth to medium-low, and cook until the bacon has delivered a portion of its fat. Add the onion, ringer pepper, and garlic and sauté until the vegetables start to relax, 5 to 10 minutes. Add the lager, espresso, grill sauce,

molasses, jalapeno (if utilizing), and cumin and stew for 10 minutes to allow the flavors to create.

2) Flush with cold water, and channel once more. Consolidate the bacon combination and the beans in a bean pot or goulash sufficiently enormous to hold them. Mix to blend.

3) When prepared to cook, start the Traeger barbecue on Smoke with the top open until the fire is set up.

Baked Beans:

Hacked grilled pork or beef brisket extra from a past flame broil meeting is an incredible expansion to these beans. In the event that you like your beans on the zesty side, add a couple alongside the bacon, onion, and ringer pepper.

Ingredients:

1) 10 cuts substantial thick-cut smoked bacon, chilly, diced
2) 1 enormous sweet onion, stripped and diced
3) 1 red or green chime pepper, stemmed, cored, and diced
4) 3 28-OUnce jars pork and beans
5) 1 Cup Traeger Regular Barbecue Sauce, or your number one grill sauce
6) 1/2 Cup pressed earthy colored sugar
7) 1/4 cup apple juice vinegar

8) 1/4 cup Worcestershire sauce
9) 3 tablespoons arranged mustard
10) 1-1/2 teaspoons ground clove

Method:

1) Put the diced bacon in a cool skillet. Turn the warmth to medium-low, and cook until the bacon has delivered a portion of its fat. Add the onion and the chime pepper and sauté until the vegetables mollify. Move to a huge blending bowl. Mix in the pork and beans, grill sauce, earthy colored sugar, vinegar, Worcestershire sauce, mustard, and clove. Fill a huge preparing container.

2) When prepared to cook, start the Traeger flame broil on Smoke with the top open until the fire is set up.

CHAPTER 8

Traeger Baked Goods and Desserts

Traeger macaroni and cheese for a crowd:

Nothing extravagant here, yet this is a remarkably fulfilling macaroni and cheddar—possibly better than Mom's—that will end up being a family top pick.

Ingredients:

1) 2 pounds elbow macaroni
2) 12 tablespoons margarine (1-1/2 Sticks), in addition to extra for buttering the skillet
3) 1/2 Cup flour
4) 1 teaspoon dry mustard
5) 1-1/2 to 2 Cups milk
6) 2 pounds Velveeta or American cheddar, cut into 1/2-INCh blocks
7) 1-1/2 Cups ground gentle cheddar
8) 2 Cups plain dry breadcrumbs
9) Salt and dark pepper
10) Paprika
11) 1 expendable aluminum broiling container, or huge warmth verification dish.

Method:

1) Bring 5 quarts of water to a bubble in an enormous stockpot over high warmth. Add 1 tablespoon of salt. Add the macaroni, and mix. Cook for 2 minutes not exactly the time suggested on] the bundle, mixing intermittently to shield the pasta from staying. The pasta will keep on cooking in the Traeger. Channel well, and move to a huge blending bowl.

2) Meanwhile, liquefy 8 tablespoons (1 Stick) of spread in a medium pot over medium warmth. Slowly add the flour and mustard, whisking continually. Keep whisking for around 2 minutes, being cautious that the blend doesn't start to brown. The margarine/flour combination will bubble. Step by step speed in 1-1/2 Cups of milk; whisk consistently until the blend is smooth. Lessen the warmth to medium-low and mix in the Velveeta, each third in turn, until all the cheddar is fused and dissolved. Add more milk if the cheddar sauce appears to be excessively thick. Season to taste with salt and pepper. Pour the cheddar sauce over the pasta and mix delicately with an elastic spatula or wooden spoon. Margarine the simmering skillet or goulash. Pour the macaroni and cheddar uniformly into the dish. Sprinkle the cheddar on top.

3) Melt the leftover 4 tablespoons of margarine in a pan. Add the breadcrumbs, and mix to

cover with spread. Spread the breadcrumbs equally over the highest point of the macaroni and cheddar. Residue delicately with paprika.

4) When prepared to cook, start the Traeger flame broil on Smoke with the cover open until the fire is set up.

5) Bake the macaroni and cheddar for 45 minutes to 60 minutes, or until the blend is hot and gurgling and the breadcrumbs are brilliant earthy colored.

Garlic Bread 1:

Watch out for this as it flames broils; bread can consume effectively—even on a Traeger!

Ingredients:

1) 1 portion Italian or French bread
2) 10 tablespoons spread (1-1/4 sticks), at room temperature
3) Garlic salt, for example, Lawry's
4) 3 tablespoons new parsley, or 1 tablespoon dried parsley

Method:

1) Using a serrated bread blade, cautiously cut the bread down the middle longwise, making two long parts. Margarine the cut sides, and sprinkle with garlic salt.

2) When prepared to cook, start the Traeger flame broil on Smoke with the cover open until the fire is set up.

3) Arrange the two bread parts on the flame broil grind, buttered sides down. Flame broil until the bread starts to brown, 10 to 12 minutes. Utilizing utensils, turn the bread over. Sprinkle it with the parsley. Move to a cutting board, and utilizing a bread blade, cut into cuts. Serve warm.

Garlic Bread 2:

It's so natural to cook garlic on your Traeger. Simply sprinkle it with olive oil, envelop it by foil, and in under 60 minutes, you'll have the genuine article for making marvellous garlic bread.

Ingredients:

1) 2 teaspoons extra-virgin olive oil
2) 10 tablespoons spread (1-1/4 sticks), at room temperature
3) Salt and newly ground dark pepper
4) 3/4 cup finely ground Parmesan cheddar
5) 3 tablespoons new parsley, or 1 tablespoon dried parsley

Method:

1) (No compelling reason to strip.) Adequately huge to wall it in. Sprinkle the olive oil over the garlic, and bring the edges of the foil up to freely wall it in.

2) When prepared to cook, start the Traeger flame broil on Smoke with the top open until the fire is set up.

3) On the off chance that making the bread promptly, don't kill the barbecue. (You can cook the garlic ahead of time, or at a past flame broil meeting.)

4) Let the garlic cool somewhat, at that point crush the sides over a little bowl to deliver the simmered garlic. Dispose of the papery husk. Add the spread and salt and pepper to taste and beat with a wooden spoon until joined. Utilizing a serrated bread blade, cautiously cut the bread into equal parts longwise, making two long parts. Spread the cut sides with the garlic margarine.

5) Increase the flame broil temperature to 400 degrees F.

6) Arrange the two bread parts on the flame broil grind, buttered sides down. Flame broil until the bread starts to brown, 10 to 12 minutes.

7) Utilizing utensils, turn the bread over. Sprinkle it uniformly with the cheddar, at that point the parsley. Flame broil for 2 minutes more to liquefy the cheddar. Move to a cutting board, and utilizing a bread blade, cut into cuts. Serve warm.

Blueberry-sour cream muffins:

Occasionally, Traeger proprietors in some northern states and Canada can scavenge for wild blueberries. Be that as it may, blueberries from the store or rancher's market in the little mollusc shell compartments—and even frozen blueberries—turn out only great in this formula. The sharp cream makes these biscuits especially delicate and clammy.

Ingredients:

1) 2 Cups flour
2) 1/2 teaspoon salt
3) 1/2 teaspoon heating pop
4) 1/2 Cup spread
5) 3/4 cup sugar, in addition to extra for the biscuit tops
6) 2 enormous eggs
7) 3/4 cup acrid cream
8) 1-1/2 teaspoons vanilla
9) 1-1/2 Cups new or frozen blueberries
10) Paper cupcake liners
11) Butter, at room temperature, for serving

Method:

1) In a little blending bowl, consolidate the flour, salt, and preparing pop; whisk. In another bowl, utilizing a wooden spoon or a blender, beat the spread and sugar until light-shaded and soft. Beat in the eggs, each in turn. Mix in the acrid cream and vanilla. Utilizing an elastic spatula, delicately crease in the blueberries.

2) Line a 12-Cup biscuit tin with the cupcake liners. Utilizing a frozen yogurt scoop or spoon, fill every biscuit cup 66% full with the hitter. Sprinkle sugar uniformly over the highest point of every biscuit.

3) When prepared to cook, start the Traeger barbecue on Smoke with the top open until the fire is set up.

4) Bake the biscuits 25 to 30 minutes, or until a toothpick embedded in the focal point of one confesses all (no uncooked player sticking to it). Turn the skillet 180 degrees partially through the preparing time. Serve warm or at room temperature with margarine, whenever wanted.

Old-Fashioned Cornbread:

It just takes a couple of moments to stir up cornbread without any preparation.

Ingredients:

1) 1 Cup universally handy flour
2) 1 Cup yellow or white cornmeal
3) 1 tablespoon sugar
4) 2 teaspoons heating powder
5) 1/2 teaspoon salt
6) 3 tablespoons margarine
7) 1 Cup milk
8) 1 enormous egg, gently beaten

Method:

1) In a blending bowl, join the flour, cornmeal, sugar, heating powder, and salt. Soften the margarine in a little pot. (Ensure the blend isn't hot or the egg will turn sour.) Add the milk-egg combination to the dry fixings and mix to join. Don't overmix. Spread the hitter uniformly in a lubed 8-or 9-inch square preparing dish or pie plate.

2) When prepared to cook, start the Traeger barbecue on Smoke with the cover open until the fire is set up.

3) Bake the cornbread until it starts to pull away from the sides of the skillet and the top is starting to brown, 25 to 35 minutes. Cut into squares (or wedges, in the event that you utilized a pie plate) for serving.

Blonde" Brownies:

This formula goes together shortly and will turn into a top choice in your Traeger dessert collection.

Ingredients:

1) Cooking splash
2) 6 tablespoons spread
3) 1 Cup stuffed earthy colored sugar
4) 1 huge egg
5) 1 teaspoon vanilla concentrate
6) 1 Cup flour
7) 1/2 teaspoon preparing powder
8) 1/8 teaspoon preparing pop
9) Pinch of salt
10) 1/2 Cup chocolate chip pieces
11) 1/2 Cup walnuts or pecans, hacked (discretionary)
12) Ice cream and jostled caramel garnish for serving

Method:

1) Coat a 9-inch glass pie plate or 8-by 8-inch glass heating dish with cooking splash.

2) Melt the spread in a medium pan over low warmth. Add the earthy colored sugar and mix with a wooden spoon until consolidated. Eliminate from the warmth and let cool marginally. (Excessively hot, and it will coagulate the egg.) Beat in the egg and vanilla. Filter the flour, preparing powder, heating pop, and salt into the earthy colored sugar combination. Mix to join. Mix in the nuts, if utilizing.

3) Spread the batter equally in the readied pie plate or container. Sprinkle with the chocolate chips.

4) When prepared to cook, start the Traeger flame broil on Smoke with the cover open until the fire is set up.

5) Starts to side of the preparing dish, turning part of the way through the cooking time. Let cool marginally, at that point cut into wedges (on the off chance that you utilized a pie plate) or squares (in the event that you utilized a rectangular dish). Serve warm with frozen yogurt and jostled caramel fixing, whenever wanted.

Easy Carrot Cake:

You can even avoid the icing completely and essentially filter powdered sugar over the cooled cake. In the event that you like, you can split the hitter between biscuit cups fixed with paper cupcake liners. Diminish time on the Traeger to 20 to 25 minutes if heating cupcakes.

Ingredients:

1) 8 huge carrots, stripped and cut into 1-INCh pieces
2) 4 eggs
3) 1 Cup vegetable oil
4) 1/2 Cup milk
5) 1 teaspoon vanilla
6) 2 Cups granulated sugar
7) 2 Cups flour
8) 2 tablespoons cocoa
9) 2 teaspoons preparing pop
10) 1/2 teaspoon salt
11) 1 Cup raisins (discretionary)
12) Solid shortening or nonstick cooking splash for the dish
13) Cream Cheese Icing (formula underneath) or powdered sugar

Method:

1) Join the carrots, eggs, oil, milk, also, vanilla and cycle until the carrots are in little pieces. Put the sugar into a huge blending bowl. Filter in the flour, cocoa, heating pop, and salt. Pour in the carrot combination, and mix until the wet and dry fixings are simply joined. Mix in the raisins, whenever wanted.

2) Grease a 9X13-inch preparing dish with shortening or splash it with cooking shower. Empty the hitter into the readied dish.

3) When prepared to cook, start the Traeger flame broil on Smoke with the cover open until the fire is set up.

4) Bake the cake for roughly 60 minutes, or until a toothpick embedded in the middle tells the truth. Turn the dish 180 degrees partially through the preparing time. Cool the cake totally on a cake rack prior to icing with Cream Cheese Icing (formula underneath) or tidying with powdered sugar.

5) Using a hand blender, consolidate 4 ounces of cream cheddar, 2-1/2 Cups powdered sugar, 3 tablespoons room-temperature spread, 1 teaspoon of vanilla, and a touch of salt. Add milk or cream varying to get the ideal consistency; beat until cushy. Ice the cooled cake.

Peach and Raspberry Crisp:

Blueberries, apples, pears, cherries, and even rhubarb function admirably in this formula. Utilize anything that's in season.

Ingredients:

1) 6 cups diced peaches
2) 8 tablespoons cold spread, cut into 1-INCh pieces
3) 1/8 teaspoon salt
4) Ice cream for serving

Method:

1) Grease a 9-or 10-INCh pie plate with cooking splash or strong shortening. In an enormous blending bowl. Mix to consolidate. Fill the readied pie plate.

2) In the bowl of a food processor, consolidate the cookies, earthy colored sugar, spread, salt, and the leftover 1/2 Cup of flour. Heartbeat until the cookies are brittle and the spread has been separated into pea-sized pieces. Spoon the garnish equally over the organic product in the pie plate.

3) When prepared to cook, start the Traeger

flame broil on Smoke with the cover open
until the fire is set up.

4) Bake the fresh until the filling is rising around
the edges of the pie plate and the fixing is
pleasantly sautéed, around 45 minutes. Serve
warm with frozen yogurt, whenever wanted.

Chocolate-Chipotle Brownies:

Chipotle chiles (smoked jalapenos) and cinnamon are
matched with a boxed brownie blend for a sweet with
a delicate however captivating kick. Whenever
wanted, serve the brownies with cinnamon or vanilla
frozen yogurt showered with chocolate sauce.

Method:

1) Prepare the brownie blend as indicated by
bundle bearings. Mix in the adobo sauce and
the cinnamon.

2) Grease a 9-by 13-inch preparing dish with
shortening or splash it with cooking shower.
Equitably spread the brownie player into the
readied skillet.

3) When prepared to cook, start the Traeger
barbecue on Smoke with the top open until the
fire is set up.

4) Bake the brownies until done, yet fudgy,
around 25 to 28 minutes, turning the dish 180

degrees part of the way through the cooking time. Let cool. Cut into squares.

Chocolate Chip Cookies:

Vinegar isn't a misprint in this formula. It softens the cookies

Ingredients:

1) 2-3/4 cups generally useful flour, in addition to extra if necessary
2) 1-1/2 teaspoons preparing pop
3) 1/2 teaspoon salt
4) 1 Cup white sugar
5) 1 Cup earthy colored sugar
6) 1 Cup strong shortening, for example, Crisco
7) 2 eggs
8) 2-1/2 teaspoons apple juice vinegar
9) 1 teaspoon vanilla
10) 2 Cups (12 ounces) chocolate chips
11) 1 Cup coarsely hacked nuts

Method:

1) Lay a bit of cooking material paper on a cookie sheet.

2) Combine the flour, heating pop, and salt in a blending bowl and mix well to consolidate.

3) Using a wooden spoon, a hand-held blender, or a stand blender, cream together the white

sugar, earthy colored sugar, and shortening. Blend in the eggs, vinegar, and vanilla. Add the flour blend to the sugar combination and join. Mix in the chocolate chips and nuts, whenever wanted.

4) The batter should be sufficiently firm—even marginally tacky—to fold into balls (about golf-ball size). In the event that excessively tacky, dust somewhat more flour over the mixture and blend in. In the event that excessively firm, add a tablespoon of water or milk, or varying in little augmentations. Orchestrate 9 balls in columns on the readied cookie sheet. Smooth the balls with the palm of your hand or the lower part of a glass.

5) When prepared to cook, start the Traeger barbecue on Smoke with the cover open until the fire is set up. Prepare the cookies for 10 to 12 minutes. Give the skillet a sharp rap on the barbecue grind prior to eliminating the cookies. This collapses them and makes them chewier. Cool the cookies on a cooling rack. Prepare the leftover cookies as coordinated previously.

Mango Chipotle Smoked and Fried Chicken Wings:

Ingredients:

1) 3 pounds chicken wings
2) 2 tablespoons avocado oil
3) 3 tablespoons Mango Chipotle Rub
4) sauce based on your personal preference

Method:

1) Spot the wings onto a rack, in a solitary layer, and put them in the ice chest short-term to dry.

2) Eliminate from the ice chest and throw in the oil. Coat generously with the Mango Chipotle Seasoning.

3) Fire up your pellet flame broil and set it to 180°.

4) Spot the wings on the barbecue and smoke for 2 hours, turning once part of the way through the smoke.

5) Eliminate the wings from the smoker, and preheat your oil to 375.

6) Drop the wings in little clumps and fry for 4-6 minutes, or until the skin is firm. The chicken

should be cooked to around 160 - 180 degrees from the long, slow smoke, however this last fry will guarantee they are cooked through too.

7) Eliminate from the oil, let channel, and afterward throw in your #1 wing sauce.

Smoked Breakfast Fatty:

Our Cheese and Hash brown Stuffed Breakfast Fatty takes firm, new has earthy colours, loads them with cheddar, at that point moves the entirety of that up inside breakfast hotdog prior to enveloping the WHOLE thing by bacon. At that point it hits the pellet flame broil until it is cooked through and the bacon is fresh for a wood-terminated breakfast greasy that you will probably remember forever!

What kinds of barbecues would you be able to use to cook this?

We have utilized essentially pellet flame broils for our smoking/barbecuing throughout the previous quite a long while. Those incorporate two or three Traeger's, a Camp Chef Woodwind, and a Louisiana Vertical Pellet Smoker as well. You can cook this on some other sort of smoker, or some other sort of barbecue over aberrant warmth. Utilize similar temperatures, or as close as you can get to it in any case, and a smoke cylinder would not damage either on the off chance that you are utilizing a propane flame broil to make this formula.

Ingredients:

1) 1-pound breakfast wiener
2) 2 cups arranged hash browns
3) 1 cup destroyed Colby jack cheddar
4) 1-pound bacon
5) 1 tablespoon rub

Method:

1) Preheat your pellet flame broil to 250°, following production line kind of flame broil, ensure you are cooking over backhanded warmth.

2) Utilizing the entire pound of bacon, make your bacon weave on top of a sheet. Adhere to these directions on the off chance that you don't know how to make a bacon weave.

3) Set out the cling wrap and pat out the morning meal wiener into around a 6x6 square.

4) Layer the hash browns and cheddar over the top and press tenderly.

5) Roll the wiener up, similar to a cinnamon move, into a log.

6) Utilizing the cling wrap, cautiously move the hotdog roll onto the bacon weave, and move off the cling wrap so it is on top of the bacon.

7) Wrap the bacon weave around the greasy, and either attach with butcher's twine to keep it together or place it cautiously on a sheet of non-stick foil (eliminating the saran wrap) and spot it on the barbecue.

8) Cook, turning intermittently until the inside temp is 165° and the bacon is fresh.

9) Eliminate, let sit for 10 minutes, and afterward cut and serve.

Tips for an ideal Breakfast Fatty

1) Breakfast fatties are pretty simple to make on the off chance that you follow some basic hints that will save you some disappointment.

2) Ensure your hash browns are cooked, yet chilly when you put them on the pork. In the event that you put hot hash browns on their it will make it harder for the entire thing to remain together.

3) Move it cautiously. You don't need it to self-destruct after it is moved up.

Traeger Butter Swim Biscuits:

These Traeger Butter Swim Biscuits will turn into an end of the week staple in your morning meal schedule. They are easy to put together and asking for a goliath pile of raspberry jam or to be transformed into the most epic of breakfast sandwiches.

Instructions to make margarine swim rolls

1) Blend the dry.
2) Dump in the wet.
3) Mix a bit.
4) Empty softened margarine into enormous square shape container.
5) Dump bread roll mixture on top.
6) Spread it. Cut it. Heat it. Eat it.

Consider the possibility that you don't have a pellet barbecue.
This formula was initially made in a customary broiler. You can follow a similar temp guides for your stove in the event that you'd preferably cook them there.

You can likewise cook these on different sorts of flame broils, simply ensure you have a vibe for the temperature control and problem areas, and turn the container varying with the goal that they don't consume.

1) Bread rolls are about the surface, and the surface is about NOT OVERMIXING THE DOUGH. So, mix it as meager as you need to, to ensure all the dry fixings are not, at this point dry toward the end.
2) Use margarine or return home
3) No margarine permitted, individuals. Simply state no.
4) Measure precisely

To do that you need to do the old, flour lighten + delicate scoop into quantifying cup + level off the estimating cup as they instructed you back in Homes on the off chance that you are mature enough (like me) to have had Home Ec.

Split them with a fork

Much the same as with an English Muffin, you will need to part these with a fork by staying a fork into them right around the roll prior to parting it in two.

The most effective method to store spread swim rolls

Spread Swim Biscuits should be put away in an impenetrable compartment to keep them from drying out or getting lifeless. On the off chance that you have extras, they'll taste better the second time around in the event that you give them a little re-heat before eating.

The air fryer or stove is the best spot for warming rolls, yet I wouldn't turn down one that did several circles around the microwave by the same token.

Serving recommendations

Actually, these rolls are wonderful served up with some margarine and a liberal scoop of Raspberry Jam. It is pretty incredible, and I'm a fan.

These likewise make GREAT breakfast sandwiches as well, so fire up that Blackstone and make a few omelettes and prepare some Traeger Bacon as well.

Or on the other hand, make an epic Smoked Breakfast Fatty, cook an egg, and make the BEST breakfast sandwich, EVER.

1) 3 tablespoons preparing powder
2) 3 tablespoons earthy colored sugar
3) 1/2 tablespoons salt

Method:

1) Preheat your Traeger to high. In a perfect world, you need it to get as near 450° as you can. Soften your spread and put in a safe spot.

2) Shower a high-sided 10x13 inch barbecue safe dish with cooking splash. Pour in the spread.

3) Pour in the bread roll player and spread tenderly and equally across the container.

4) Utilizing a seat scrubber or metal spatula that has been covered in margarine, cut the rolls into 12-15 squares, letting a little softened spread summary into the cuts in the middle of the different rolls.

5) In the event that you have a top rack, place the container on the top rack of the flame broil. Lower part of your bread rolls by altering a huge rectangular cake dish on the flame broil

meshes and afterward putting your bread rolls in addition.

6) Heat for 25-30 minutes, or until the bread rolls are raised and the tops are brilliant earthy colored. Pivot the dish partially through cooking for best outcomes.

Smoked Black Cod Dip:

Smokey, and amazing to spread on your #1 saltine or toasted round of roll.

Smoked Black Cod Dip Shopping List

1) Cream cheddar
2) Acrid cream
3) Lemon
4) Garlic powder
5) Onion powder
6) Paprika
7) Green onion
8) Dark sesame seeds

Step by step instructions to make smoked fish plunge

1) Utilize the most excellent smoked fish you can get. It makes a difference and is the primary flavor in the plunge, so don't hold back!

2) Put all the fixings aside from the paprika, green onion, and dark sesame seeds into an enormous bowl and mix until they are equally joined.

Are there any replacements you can make here?

1) You can substitute plain yogurt for the harsh cream in the event that you'd like. It shouldn't affect the flavor or surface of the final product adversely.

2) You can likewise utilize some lemon squeeze rather than lemon zing in the event that you are when there's no other option.

3) I've never taken a stab at subbing in lower-fat cream cheddar, yet I additionally tend the incline toward my dairy full fat so I am certainly one-sided in such manner.

4) Some other replacements, let me know how it goes! I generally urge individuals to try and change things as indicated by their own preferences around here.

Ingredients:
1) 1 cup cream cheddar, mollified
2) 1/2 cup sharp cream
3) 12 ounces smoked Black Cod
4) 1 teaspoon new lemon zing
5) 1 teaspoon onion powder
6) 1/2 teaspoon garlic powder
7) 1/4 teaspoon dark pepper
8) 1/4 teaspoon paprika
9) 2 tablespoons slashed green onions
10) 1 teaspoon dark sesame seeds

Method:
1) Combine all the fixings aside from the paprika, green onions, and sesame seeds.

2) Chill for 2-3 hours.

3) Top with the held fixings and present with your #1 wafers or toasted loaf adjusts!

Smoked Black Cod:

This delightful Smoked Black Cod Recipe is dry tenderized prior to being gradually smoked on the pellet flame broil. Ideal for a Smokey expansion to a charcuterie board, or blended into a delicious smoked cod plunge.

Simple Smoked Black Cod
We love smoked fish around here, yet generally, we will in general adhere to our many Smoked Salmon Recipes, or when we're truly fortunate we make smoked trout.

What is Black Cod?

Dark cod is otherwise called Sablefish, Butterfish, Coalfish, Alaskan Cod, and a few other lesser-known nicknames. The bounty of names for this rich, high-oil fish is because of its notoriety in endless territories of the world.

It can really be difficult to find in the US because of the colossal ubiquity of this fish in Japan. Check your nearby fish market or extravagant supermarket for accessibility, or befriend an angler.

Instructions to smoke Black Cod

1) Brackish water the fish.
2) Flush the fish.
3) Dry the fish.
4) Let the fish build up the pellicle.
5) Smoke the fish.
6) Eat up the fish.

Instructions to store Smoked Sablefish

Like any home-smoked fish, this should be speedily wrapped and put away in the ice chest once it falls off the smoker. We like to enclose by saran wrap and afterward store in a baggie or other sealable stockpiling holder.

It will save for 7-10 days whenever put away appropriately, however I suggest vacuum-fixing and freezing.

Ingredients:

1) 1/2 pounds Black Cod filets
2) 1/4 cup fit salt
3) 1/4 cup earthy colored sugar

4) 1 teaspoon onion powder
5) 1/2 teaspoon garlic powder

Method:

1) To start with, wash your fish off with cold water and wipe off.
2) Put all your dry fixings into a little bowl and blend   well.

3) Lay your fish filets out on an enormous cutting board or some other spotless, level surface.
4) Sprinkle the dry salt water fixings onto the fish. Ensure all sides of the fish are equally covered with it.
5) Cover the fish in cling wrap and spot in the ice chest for 3-4 hours. Well, the more it brackish waters, the saltier it will be.
6) Remove the fish from the cooler, open up, and wash the salt water off of the fish.
7) Wipe the fish off, place on a cookie sheet and set it back into the cooler for 3-4 hours so the pellicle can shape.
8) Start your smoker and set it to 175 degrees Fahrenheit.
9) Spot your fish on the barbecue and let smoke for 3-4 hours.
10) Pull the fish from the barbecue, and put it in the ice chest to chill for an hour prior to saving.

Grill and Chill Shrimp Cocktail:

We made this simple shrimp mixed drink on our pellet barbecue, yet any kind of flame broil would work here. I lean toward my pellet flame broils since I think wood fire does supernatural things to fish, and shrimp particularly, however don't let the absence of a pellet barbecue shield you from making this.

Barbecue and Chill Shrimp Cocktail Shopping List

1) 1-pound kind sized shrimp
2) salt
3) onion powder
4) garlic powder
5) olive oil
6) mixed drink sauce

Purchase the huge shrimp. The greater they are, the more probable you are to NOT overcook them.

Try not to overcook them. Overcooked shrimp is rubbery and not a thing that anybody will be keeping in touch with home about. Indeed, even large shrimp will be done in a short time or less, much of the time.

Ensure there is an ideal opportunity to chill. Shrimp for shrimp mixed drink should be cold, so don't avoid that part!

Ingredients:

1) 1-pound uncooked U-20 shrimp
2) 1 teaspoon onion powder
3) 1 teaspoon garlic powder

4) tablespoon olive oil
5) 1 teaspoon salt

Method:
1) Pre-heat your pellet flame broil to 350 degrees Fahrenheit.
2) Spot your shrimp into a medium bowl and wash altogether.
3) Put them onto paper towels, and wipe off.
4) Set the shrimp back into the bowl and add all the dry fixings and the olive oil.
5) Blend by throwing the shrimp in the bowl until they are uniformly covered.
6) Spot the shrimp straightforwardly onto the pre-warmed barbecue surface.
7) Close the top to the flame broil and let cook for 10 minutes.
8) Pull the shrimp from the barbecue and spread them onto a cookie sheet.
9) Chill for one hour prior to presenting with mixed drink sauce.

Smoked Tri-Tip Recipe:

This Smoked Tri-Tip Recipe is covered with a striking Roasted Garlic Rub prior to being opposite singed on our pellet barbecue. This is one of the simplest beef dishes to make, and one of the greatest as well!

Traeger Smoked Tri-Tip Recipe

The tri-tip is one of those dishes that many individuals, shockingly, have never made. Is anything but a cut that is included at numerous eateries, at any rate that I've been to, and I didn't have my first taste until I was very much into my 30's and had been making a plunge into the grill and smoking world for quite a while.

We began to hear increasingly more about how stunning tri-tip is, and since we are regularly discovered scrutinizing the meat division in Costco, where they will in general convey these meals, we chose to give it a shot.

The most effective method to invert burn tri-tip on a Traeger Pellet Grill

There are numerous approaches to do this, and do it well, this is only the one that we like the best.

1) Coat generously with rub.

2) Spot on the barbecue and let it smoke for an hour and a half.

3) Pull the meal from the barbecue and tent with foil. Wrench the barbecue up as high as it will go.

4) Set the meal back on the barbecue once it is pre-warmed and allowed it to cook until it arrives at your ideal degree of doneness. As far as we might be concerned, that is 120°.

5) 1 tri-tip beef broil

6) Simmered Garlic Blend (or a mix of garlic powder, onion powder, paprika, salt, and pepper)

7) Preheat your pellet barbecue to 175°.

8) While the barbecue is warming, remove your meal from the refrigerator and coat generously with the rub.

9) Spot the meat on the barbecue and let cook for an hour and a half at 175°.

10) Eliminate to a plate and tent with foil. Turn the warmth on the pellet barbecue up to high, and let it preheat once more.

11) Whenever it is warmed at most extreme temps (as a rule around 400-450°), place the dish back on the barbecue and keep on cooking until the interior temperature comes to the "pull at" temp that you like.

Traeger T-Bone Grilled Steak Recipe:

This epic Reverse-Seared T-Bone Steak is a 2-inch-thick steak that is gradually smoked to a cool 115° prior to being tossed on our Blackstone frying pan that is bursting hot and burning the two sides to shape the ideal steak hull and a medium-uncommon 125° focus. After the rest, it'll be as near amazing as it can get!

Ingredients:
1) 2-pound T-bone steak
2) salt and pepper

Method:
1) Preheat your pellet barbecue or smoker to 200°. Spot the steak on and let it cook until they arrive at 115° interior temperature.

2) Eliminate from the flame broil and generously salt and pepper the steaks. Preheat a gas frying pan or cast-iron skillet over medium-high warmth, and set out a touch of oil in the container or on the frying pan.

3) Spot the steak on and burn for 1-2 minutes on each side.

4) Let rest, covered, for 5 minutes prior to cutting.

Smoked Teriyaki Beef Jerky

Beef jerky is one of my number one thing to make at home on our pellet flame broils. There's simply no correlation between what you can make at home and what you can purchase in the store.

Our unique Traeger Beef Jerky has been an immense hit, both in our home and in huge numbers of yours too, and we believe you will cherish this one similarly so much.

What cut of beef would it be advisable for you to use for this jerky?

Since we needed to make teriyaki beef jerky sticks this time around, we needed to utilize meat that could undoubtedly be cut into slight strips while as yet holding their shape.

Cutting WITH the grain likewise implies that when you nibble into the completed item you'll be gnawing pieces against the increase, making for the ideal chomp

Teriyaki Jerky Sticks shopping list

1) flank steak
2) soy sauce
3) earthy colored sugar
4) pineapple juice
5) oil
6) garlic
7) garlic, onion, and ginger powder
8) sriracha
9) apple juice vinegar

Combine the marinade fixings.
1) Marinate those sticks.

2) Dry those sticks.
3) Smoke them at 160-180° for 3-4 hours.
4) Attempt to make them last over a day or two on the off chance that you have youngsters.

Ingredients:
1) 4 pounds flank steak
2) 1/2 cup soy sauce
3) 1/2 cup earthy colored sugar
4) 1 cup pineapple juice
5) 1/3 cup oil
6) 1 tablespoon minced garlic
7) 1/2 teaspoon garlic powder
8) 2 teaspoons onion powder
9) 3 tablespoons sriracha
10) 1 teaspoon powdered ginger
11) 1/3 cup apple juice vinegar

Method:
1) Consolidate the marinade fixings and split between two huge gallon-sized baggies. Uniformly disseminate the meat between the two baggies, pound them around to completely cover the meat, and put in the cooler for 24 hours to marinate.

2) Preheat your pellet flame broil to 160-180°.

3) Channel off and dry the jerky sticks. Splash jerky racks with cooking shower and afterward place the sticks across the racks, ensuring they are not contacting.

4) The more you smoke them the drier they will be. The drier they are, the more they'll last.

5) Eliminate from the smoker and store it in the ice chest.

Traeger Eggnog Cheesecake Recipe:

Custom made Traeger Eggnog Cheesecake is a straightforward all-flavor occasional treat that is basic, exemplary, and would be a star on any sweet table.

Ingredients:
1) 7 graham saltines, squashed
2) 3 TBSP spread, liquefied
3) 2 - 8 oz bundles cream cheddar, room temperature
4) 3/4 cup white sugar
5) 1/2 cup egg nog
6) 2 tablespoons dull rum
7) 1/2 TBSP vanilla concentrate
8) 2 TBSP flour
9) 2 eggs
10) cinnamon

Method:
1) Preheat your pellet flame broil to ~325 degrees.

2) Blend liquefied spread and graham wafer pieces together well. Press into a 8 inch pie plate.

3) Blend cream cheddar and sugar for 1 moment

on medium, or until all around consolidated. Include egg no, rum, vanilla, and flour. Blend an extra moment. Include eggs and heartbeat 2-3 times. Complete the process of blending in the eggs by hand until the whites are consolidated. Don't overmix!

4) Empty cheesecake player into arranged outside. Spot your cheesecake inside the pellet flame broil on a top rack. Top rack, alter a huge cake container with high sides or spot another rack on top of the base rack to make some extra space between the fire and the cake.

5) Heat at 325 for 60-75 minutes, or until the sides are generally set and the center is still marginally jiggly. Cool on the counter for 1 hour prior to moving to the ice chest to get done with chilling for at least 3-4 hours.

Traeger Halibut with Parmesan:

Our Traeger Halibut with Parmesan Crust was SO natural, took only 20 minutes to make, and was effectively one of my number one bits of halibut I've had the entire year.

Ingredients:
1) ½ cup Parmesan cheddar, ground or destroyed
2) ¼ cup salted spread, mollified
3) 1 tablespoon mayonnaise
4) 1 tablespoon sharp cream

5) 3 tablespoons hacked chives
6) 2 pounds skinless halibut filets

Method:

1) Preheat your pellet flame broil to 375° after manufacturing plant headings.

2) Cover a flame broil safe heating sheet with material paper, and spot the halibut on top.

3) Combine the garnish fixings and spread equitably across the skinless halibut filets.

4) Flame broil for 15-20 minutes, or until the fish drops effectively with a fork.

5) Sear for 1-2 minutes whenever wanted to brown the parmesan covering.

Traeger Banana Bread:

This Traeger Banana Bread takes my exemplary harsh cream banana bread and moves it to the Traeger pellet barbecue for a provincial, wood-kissed flavour that draws out the pleasantness of the banana in the most ideal manner. This simple formula has been adjusted extraordinarily for your pellet flame broil, so whether it is the stature of summer or late in the fall, if your barbecue is available and ready to be started up you can have incredible banana bread. My banana bread formula has harsh cream in the blend and incorporates a twirl of cinnamon sugar that is unquestionably not discretionary.

Pellet Grill Banana Bread shopping list

1) Earthy colored bananas
2) Flour
3) Sugar (white and earthy colored)
4) Vanilla
5) Eggs
6) Canola oil
7) Sharp cream
8) Preparing pop
9) Cinnamon

Why utilize earthy coloured bananas?

Bananas improve as they age as the starch goes to sugar in the natural product. Notwithstanding, the surface endures once they begin to turn out to be more earthy coloured than yellow. These make earthy coloured bananas the ideal expansion to your prepared merchandise. Sweet, delicate, and scrumptious.

Earthy coloured bananas around and are urgent for banana bread, you can feel free to toss in your yellow bananas.

The most effective method to make banana bread

I love this bread. It is nearly cake-like, truth be told, and would be ideal for a spread of cream cheddar icing. We ordinarily serve it with a pot of salted margarine or the cinnamon spread underneath.

Banana bread is one of my number one prepared merchandise to make since it is SO natural, and you simply toss ALL of the fixings into a blending bowl and blend for several minutes.

There's no filtering. No dirtying three distinct dishes to ensure you can blend wet fixings, filter dry ones, and the entirety of that stuff.

I love preparing, however once in a while it is overpowering with all the dishes and how specific you as a rule must be with the entirety of the means. I can prepare that way, however I must be in the correct mind-set for it. This formula is a no brainer. Simply measure, put it across the board bowl, and blend it up. So straightforward!

The ideal spread for banana bread

At the point when you have a warm portion of banana bread that you've quite recently pulled off the barbecue, right now is an ideal opportunity to prepare a dish of this cinnamon spread.

I utilized 2 tablespoons of Spice ology's Apple Cinnamon mix and blended it in with 1/2 cup of salted margarine. It is an ideal blend in with the sweet banana bread.

Any of that and don't have any desire to hold back to arrange it, you can stir up a little clump of cinnamon sugar spread all things considered. Simply blend 1/2 teaspoon cinnamon with 1/2 cup of margarine and 1/3 cup of honey, or to taste. You'll locate a fair compromise.

Replacements and increases

Similarly, as with the majority of my plans, don't hesitate to play with this one as well. You can substitute equivalent measures of yogurt. Something like Noosa or another full-fat yogurt would be ideal. I haven't attempted it with a sans fat Greek yogurt so I can't vouch there.

In the event that you're not into cinnamon, you can skirt that as well.

Like nuts? Blend some hacked pecans or walnuts into the hitter and go insane.

Need a Brule top? Sprinkle some crude sugar over everything before you hear it.

I haven't tried this with any san's gluten anything, so if that is a need of yours, I'd discover a formula exceptionally intended for without gluten flours and adjust that one for the flame broil as opposed to attempting to make this formula sans gluten.

Tips for heating in your Traeger

A pellet barbecue is fundamentally a major wood-terminated outside broiler, however preparing in it needs a couple of exceptional contemplations to remember.

<u>Utilize the top rack</u>

Prepared merchandise and dishes tend to scotch on the base once in a while. It'll make some invite division between the fire and your container to help forestall that.

Ingredients:
   1) 4 extra ready bananas
   2) 4 enormous eggs
   3) 1/2 tablespoons vanilla
   4) 1 cup canola oil
   5) 1 cup harsh cream

6) 1 cup white sugar
7) 1 cup dim earthy colored sugar
8) 3 cups flour
9) 2 teaspoons heating pop
10) 2/3 cup white sugar
11) 1 teaspoon cinnamon

Method:

1) Preheat your Traeger to 350 degrees adhering to industrial facility guidelines.

2) Blend the entirety of the bread fixings together (NOT the Cinnamon Topping) for 2-3 minutes utilizing a blender.

3) Empty portion of the player into a readied Bundt dish. Join the cinnamon and sugar and sprinkle half over the player. Cover with the remainder of the hitter, and spread delicately if fundamental. Sprinkle on the remainder of the cinnamon sugar beating.

4) Prepare on the top rack (or on the off chance that you don't have a rack, heat on top of a reversed rectangular cake dish to make some extra space between the fire and the nourishment) for around 60 minutes, turning part of the way through. Cook until a toothpick comes out with soggy morsels. The specific time will fluctuate dependent on numerous elements.

5) Watch cautiously! Your bread may take somewhat less time, or somewhat more time contingent upon the barbecue and your

particular container.

Meatball Stuffed Shells:

Meatball Stuffed Shells is a simple dish of my number one solace food, and utilizing your pellet barbecue to do the preparing not just adds a touch of wood-discharged flavour yet in addition shields you from warming up your kitchen in the hotter months as well.

Stuffed shells are one of my #1 dinners, however commonly you'll see them loaded down with cheddar. That form is astonishing, yet I needed to have a go at something somewhat extraordinary. We took my commonly meatball blend, less the breadcrumbs and bread, and put it directly into standard bubbled enormous shells prior to getting finished off with marinara and bountiful measures of cheddar and heated off in your pellet barbecue. I incline toward beef for meatballs, or a blend will in general go ALL beef, and get a lean assortment that is 90/10 or 95/5, in the event that you can discover it.

We get the entirety of our meat these days from Butcher Box! Their ground beef tastes astonishing, is grass-taken care of, and is adequately lean to not give up overflowing measures of oil without giving up flavour.

Ingredients:
1) 24 huge shells
2) 2 pounds lean ground beef (90/10 and no more)
3) 2 teaspoons Italian flavoring mix
4) 1/2 teaspoon garlic powder

5) 1/2 teaspoon onion powder
6) 1 teaspoon salt
7) 1/2 teaspoon pepper
8) 1 egg, beaten
9) 8 cups marinara sauce
10) 2 cups destroyed mozzarella cheddar
11) 2 cups destroyed Italian mix cheese24 enormous shells
12) 2 pounds lean ground beef (90/10 and no more)
13) 2 teaspoons Italian flavoring mix
14) 1/2 teaspoon garlic powder
15) 1/2 teaspoon onion powder
16) 1 teaspoon salt
17) 1/2 teaspoon pepper
18) 1 egg, beaten
19) 8 cups marinara sauce
20) 2 cups destroyed mozzarella cheddar
21) 2 cups destroyed Italian mix cheddar

Method:

1) Pre-heat your pellet barbecue or broiler to 350°.

2) Standard heat up the noodles (which means, cook them for a large portion of the called-for time) in very much salted water. Eliminate and flush with cold water.

3) Combine the ground beef, Italian flavoring, garlic and onion powder, salt, pepper, and the beaten egg well.

4) Fill each shell with meat combination and spot

them into an enormous high-sided rectangular preparing dish (9x12 or 10x13 works extraordinary.) If you have overabundance meat, make a few meatballs and thud them into the container as well.

5) Spot the dish into the pre-warmed barbecue or stove. In the case of utilizing a flame broil, place it on the top rack. Top rack, get some extra detachment between the fire and your dish by setting it on top of another modified high-sided rectangular cake container.

6) Let prepare for 30-45 minutes, or until the cheddar is softened and the inner temperature of the meat comes to in any event 165°.

7) Eliminate from flame broil/stove, let sit for 10 minutes, and serve hot with some new cut basil on top (whenever wanted).

Pizza Crust Recipe:

Ingredients:

1) 0.47 L warm water (110F - 115F)
2) 59 milliliters olive oil
3) Two bundles yeast
4) 1 2/5 L generally useful flour
5) 9 9/10 milliliters of salt yellow cornmeal

Method:

Evidence yeast with support in warm water. Blend yeast, water, and olive oil mix in flour 1 cup at once. Turn out onto the floured surface, ply until smooth, 5 to 7 moments, including flour as necessary. The batter will be delicate. A spot in an oiled bowl, going to cover all sides. Punch down and let rest 15 mins. Partition down the middle a, press out into two 12-inch round pizza dish or 10x15x1 skillet or 1 of each. Sprinkled with yellow cornmeal (prevents outside layer from staying).

Pizza Dough (Bread Machine) Recipe:

Ingredients:

1) 1 cup water PLUS"PLUS" signifies this fixing notwithstanding the one on the following line, regularly with separated employments
2) Two tablespoons water
3) Two tablespoons oil
4) 3 cups bread flour
5) One teaspoon sugar
6) One teaspoon salt
7) 2 1/2 teaspoons dynamic dry yeast

Method:

Spot ingredients in the dish all together recorded or as coordinated per machine directions. Select the white mixture cycle. Makes two 12-inch standard outside layers or one 16-inch dish hull. Top with necessary fixings and prepare at 400°F for 18-20 minutes or until the covering is light darker.

Pizza Dough and Sauce Recipe:

Ingredients:

1) 3/4 tablespoon yeast
2) 1 1/2 cup water
3) 1 1/2 teaspoon salt
4) Three tablespoons oil
5) 4 cups flour
6) 6 ounces would tomato be able to glue
7) 1/2 cup wine or water
8) One teaspoon oregano
9) One teaspoon salt
10) One tablespoon sugar
11) One tablespoon vegetable oil or olive oil
12) 1 1/2 tablespoon parmesan cheddar

Method:

Break down yeast in water (You can include a touch of sugar). Mix in salt, oil, and half of the flour. Continuously include remaining flour, blending great. Work 8-10 minutes or until smooth and flexible. Spot in a lobed bowl and let ascend until twofold (1/2 60 minutes). Punch down and let rise again until twofold.

Punch down and isolate. Work out on pizza dish. Top with pizza sauce and fixings. Heat at 400 for 20-25 minutes. Pizza Sauce: Mix all ingredients, mixing great (You can likewise include a couple of sprinkles of garlic powder if you need). Top with meats, cheddar, and different fixings.

Polenta Pizza Crust Recipe:

Ingredients:

1) One tablespoon Active dry yeast
2) One tablespoon Barley malt extricate
3) 1 cup of warm water
4) 3/4 cup semolina
5) 1 cup unbleached generally useful flour
6) 3/4 cup polenta/corn dinner
7) One teaspoon salt
8) Three tablespoons additional virgin olive oil

Method:

In a considerable bowl or electric blender, break up the yeast and grain malt in warm water. Include the semolina, flour, polenta, salt, and olive oil. Join well. Massage the batter until it is sparkly and smooth, including flour varying. Spot the batter in a softly oiled bowl, spread with cling wrap, and let ascend until multiplied, around 2 hours.

At the point when the batter has risen, punch down and turn out to a large circle and move to a preparing sheet or pizza skillet. Top with any favored fixing and prepare in a preheated 425F grill for 20 - 25 minutes. This is acceptably topped with broiled veggies.

Pourable Pizza Crust Recipe

Ingredients:

1) Three tablespoons Instant High-Active dry yeast
2) Warm water (110 degrees F) (just enough to break up the dynamic yeast)
3) 7 pounds All-reason or bread flour
4) One bundle (1 lb. 2 1/2 oz.) Instant nonfat dry milk
5) 8 3/4 ounces Sugar
6) 1 1/4 teaspoon salt
7) 1/8 cup Olive oil
8) Cornmeal

Method:

Break up dry yeast in warm water. =20 Let stand 5 minutes. Spot flour, milk, sugar, and salt in the blender bowl. Utilizing a whip, mix on low speed for 8 minutes. Include disintegrated yeast and oil. Mix on medium speed for 10 minutes. The player will be uneven. Oil three sheet container (18" X26" X1").

Sprinkle each dish with 1 oz (around 3 Tbsp) cornmeal. Pour or spread 3 lb 6 oz (1/2 quart) player into each container. Let represent 25 minutes. Prepare until the outside layer is set: Conventional Oven: 475 degrees F, 10 minutes. Convection Oven: 425 degrees F, 7 minutes. Top each prebaked outside with wanted garnish. Prepare until warmed through, and cheddar is dissolved: Conventional Oven: 475 degrees F, 10-15 minutes. Convection Oven: 425 degrees F, 5 minutes.

Delicate Pizza Dough Recipe:

Ingredients:

1) 3 cups bread flour
2) 7/8 cup warm water
3) One tablespoon vegetable shortening (Crisco)
4) One teaspoon dynamic dry yeast
5) One teaspoon salt
6) 1/2 teaspoon sugar

Method:

In an unflinching stand blender fitted with mix get, join the water, shortening, yeast, and sugar. Blend absolutely until the yeast has wholly isolated. Join flour and salt. Blend on low until the more significant part of the flour and water has blended, by then keep controlling for 10 minutes. The mix will be free and crude from the earliest starting point and will finally structure a firm ball. There ought to be no unpleasant flour or pieces staying in the bowl.

The hitter will be, to some degree, dry and thick. Perceive the mixing ball into a gigantic bowl and spread unequivocally with stick wrap. Let the player ascend for 24 hours in the cooler before utilizing it. You should observe that I can't over-stress the centrality of a 24-HOUR rising time since it is colossal so the mix will build up its engraving surface and, much more in a general sense, its captivating flavor! Put forth an attempt not to dodge this development!

Preheat your broiler to 500 F around one hour before you hope to warm the pizza. Turn the mix out onto a large surface and development with flour. Utilizing a fantastic moving pin, turn the hitter out flimsy to plot a 24-inch or more prominent circle. On the occasion that you're utilizing a shaper pizza dish (prescribed), dust the skillet tenderly with flour, place the hitter in the compartment, and dock. Utilize the moving pin to trim off the abundance mix hanging over the sides of the dish. Cook the pizza genuinely on a pizza stone (not utilizing a holder), by then recognize the mix on a cleaned pizza-strip, dock, and overlay the edge more than 1-INCH straightforwardly around and pound it up to layout a raised lip or edge.

Next, precook the outside layer for 4 minutes before including any sauce or fixings. Expel the outside layer from the flame broil and pop any large air pockets that may have shaped.

Fuse your sauce, wrecked mozzarella cheddar, and your supported fixings. Keep warming, turning the skillet for the most part through with the target that it cooks unbiasedly, until the covering is adequately caramelized and fresh, around 10 to 15 minutes. Expel the pizza from the flame broil and slide the pizza out of the cooking holder onto a large wire cooling rack or cutting board. Award to cool for 5 minutes before moving to a serving dish. This development permits the outside layer to remain fresh while it cools; in any case, they got steam will release up the edge. Right when cold, utilize a pizza shaper to cut the pie into pieces and appreciate it!

Entire Wheat Pizza Crust Recipe

Ingredients:

1) 1 1/4 cup warm water
2) 1/4 teaspoon salt - discretionary
3) Two tablespoons nectar or sugar
4) 2 cups usually necessary flour - isolated
5) 1 cup entire wheat flour
6) Two teaspoons dynamic dry yeast
7) One tablespoon cornmeal

Method:

Measure carefully, setting all ingredients aside from cornmeal in bread machine skillet all together directed by proprietor's manual. Program mix cycle setting; press start. Expel mix from bread machine holder; let rest 2 to 3 minutes. Pat and gently stretch mix into a 14-to 15-INCH circle. Sprinkle 14-inch pizza compartment with non-stick cooking shower; sprinkle with cornmeal, at whatever point required. Press hitter into the dish. Follow adorn and preparing headings for specific plans. One thick 14-INCH outside layer is eight servings

In a large pot, delicately sauté the onion in the oil until direct. Add the tomatoes and bring them to the air pocket. When stewing, fuse the tomato puree, the vinegar, and sugar. Stew for an entire hour, utilizing a wooden spoon to disconnect any tomato pieces. On the off chance that the sauce, regardless of everything, has bits of tomato, experience a strainer before constraining and dealing with in the cooler for to around fourteen days. Spread pathetically on pizza, use over pasta with a ground, robust, hard cheddar, or use as a base for continuously complex meat sauces for pasta.

Fundamental Pizza Sauce Recipe:

Ingredients:

1) 35 ounces canned entire tomatoes
2) One teaspoon basil
3) One clove garlic, stripped and squashed
4) Two tablespoons tomato stick
5) salt and pepper - to taste

Method:

Pour the substance of the tomato can into a 2-quart, extensive non-aluminum holder and coarsely pound the tomatoes with a fork. Consolidate the herbs, garlic, tomato glue, salt, and pepper. Bring to an air pocket over medium warmth, stirring to blend the seasonings.

Exactly when the sauce starts to bubble, turn the sparkle to low and keep up the sauce at a delicate stew. Cook, revealed, stirring from time to time, for at any rate 15 minutes and an imperative of 60 minutes.

Firehouse Pizza Sauce Recipe:

Ingredients:

1) 1 (6 ounces) would tomato have the choice to stick
2) 3/4 cup warm water (110 degrees F/45 degrees C)
3) Three tablespoons ground Parmesan cheddar
4) One teaspoon minced garlic
5) One tablespoon Honey or Splenda on the off chance that you may require low carb
6) One teaspoon anchovy stick (discretionary)
7) 3/4 teaspoon onion powder

8) 1/4 teaspoon dried oregano
9) 1/4 teaspoon dried marjoram
10) 1/4 teaspoon dried basil
11) 1/4 teaspoon ground dull pepper
12) 1/8 teaspoon cayenne pepper
13) 1/8 teaspoon dried red pepper chips

Method:

In a little bowl, harden tomato stick, water, Parmesan cheddar, garlic, Splenda, anchovy stick, onion powder, oregano, marjoram, basil, ground diminish pepper, cayenne pepper, red pepper pieces, and salt; unite, disconnecting any heaps of cheddar. Spread over pizza players and plan pizza varying.

Mince onion and garlic. Sauté in olive oil until onion is transparent and delicate. Add the rest of the ingredients to skillet and stew for 15-20 minutes. Makes enough sauce for two pizzas. Additionally, makes a beguiling sauce for breadsticks and calzones. Slash onion and garlic, microwave for five minutes (discard this progression if you don't have a microwave; it isn't basic; however, it makes the sauce faster to cook). Move to the pan, include tomato puree and mix. Include tinned tomatoes. Season, bring to bubble, and stew for around 15-20 minutes until it has diminished to a jammy consistency. For flavoring, I utilize salt, crisply processed dark pepper, Worcestershire sauce, and a herb, new basil if I have it, or dried Italian flavoring.

Reverse-Seared Flat Iron Steak Recipe:

Our Reverse-Seared Flat Iron Steak Recipe takes excellent level iron steaks and smokes them on a pellet flame broil prior to being singed at high warmth on a gas frying pan or in a cast iron container on the burner, for a definitive in steak outside layer.

Ingredients:
1) 6 level iron steaks
2) salt and pepper

Method:
1) Preheat your pellet flame broil or smoker to 200°. Spot the steaks on and let them cook until they arrive at 115° inside temperature.

2) Eliminate from the barbecue and generously salt and pepper the steaks. Preheat a gas frying pan or cast-iron dish over medium-high warmth, and set out a touch of oil in the container or on the frying pan.

3) Spot the steaks on, and singe for 1-2 minutes on each side.

4) Let rest, covered, for 5 minutes prior to cutting.

Tequila Lime Smoked Shredded Beef:

Smoked Shredded Beef Tacos are a significant piece, without help from anyone else, however toss in a braising fluid spiked with tequila and the entire thing goes in a newly singed puffy taco shell? Don't worry about it.

Shopping List
In the event that you don't have something that this requires, the formula itself is pretty sympathetic. Locate your nearest hoodwink and get down to business.

1) Toss cook
2) Spice ology Chile Lime preparing
3) SPG
4) beef stock
5) tequila (use code "DRIZLYDEAL" for $5 off!)
6) El Pato Jalapeno pureed tomatoes
7) Limes
8) Maseca (moment corn masa flour)
9) vegetable oil

Step by step instructions to make smoked destroyed beef tacos

The cycle is simple, despite the fact that the process can't be rushed, and you have a great deal of choices as well.

1) Rub
2) Smoke

3) Braise
4) Shred
5) Rub it

To start with, rub the meat. I utilized a mix of SPG (salt, pepper, garlic) and Spice ology's Chile lime mix.

Smoke it

Next, smoke it! We utilized our pellet barbecue, yet you could utilize a stick burner or an electric smoker if that is the thing that you have around. You can even utilize a smoke tube in a charcoal or gas barbecue if that is the thing that you have.

Braise it

When the meat gets an opportunity to smoke for a couple of hours, the time has come to braise the meat. In this formula, I utilized my Instant Pot. In the electric weight cooker under high tension, it took an hour with a 15-minute normal constrain delivery to get it there. I generally start with a 30-minute high-compel cook and afterward test it to perceive how close it is. Various cuts of meat cook at various rates, and it likewise relies upon how far along the meat got during the smoke parcel.

Instant Pot you can likewise utilize the broiler, a stewing pot, or even proceed with things on your smoker. You'll need to run it at around 300-325°, firmly covered, until the dish arrives at 204-205° and is fork-delicate.

Shred it

When the meal is finished braising, it'll be fork delicate. That is the way you realize it is finished. Shred the beef in your braising fluid, and stew to decrease the fluid a piece.

Ingredients:
1) 4-pound beef throw broil
2) 3 tablespoons chile margarita mix
3) 2 tablespoons salt, pepper, garlic mix
4) 2 cups beef stock
5) 4 ounces silver tequila
6) 2 limes, squeezed
7) 2 jars El Pato Jalapeno pureed tomatoes
8) 2 1/2 cups masa harina
9) 1/2 teaspoons salt
10) 1 2/3 cups warm water
11) oil for fricasseeing

Method:
1) Preheat your pellet barbecue to 200-225°.

2) Rub the meat with the rub fixings, and put it into the smoker, straightforwardly on the barbecue.

3) Following three hours, place into your Instant pot. A huge heating dish appropriate for braising will do. A Dutch stove, high-sided dispensable foil dish, or a huge rectangular bit of plated stoneware would work moreover.

4) Pour over the braising fluid fixings, place the cover on the pot, and set to an hour, high weight. If not utilizing an Instant Pot, increment the warmth on your barbecue, broiler, or moderate cooker to be around 325°. Firmly cover your preparing dish to keep all the juices and dampness inside the heating

dish.

5) When the Instant Pot cycle is done, let the weight discharge normally for at any rate 15 minutes prior to venting the abundance and opening it up. The dish should be fork-delicate. In the event that it isn't, set it back in the pot and close it up for an additional 15-minute cycle.

6) If not utilizing an Instant Pot, simply cook the dish until it is fork-delicate and shred able. The measure of time it will take differs significantly relying upon your specific bit of meat, the climate you are cooking in, and so forth I'd by and by begin checking at around 2 1/2 - 3 hours and keep on checking each 30-45 minutes until it was done.

7) Shred the beef, eliminating any enormous pieces of fat or cartilage. Keep the meat in the braising fluid to keep it damp.

8) Start the shells around 30 minutes before the beef is done cooking by combining the entirety of the Puffy Taco Shell fixings until it is smooth and completely consolidated, and preheating 3 creeps of oil in a medium-sized pot or fryer to 375°.

9) Fold the batter into 12 similarly estimated balls. Take a huge ziplock and cut open along the two side creases. Leave the base crease unblemished. Spot this into your tortilla press or onto your counter, and either press or fold

the tortilla ball into a hover that is around 5-6" across and 1/8 inch in thickness.

10) Cautiously drop the tortilla into the hot oil and let it puff up. It should take under 30 seconds.

11) Utilizing two arrangements of utensils, flip over the puffy tortilla and promptly push down in the focal point of the taco shell and lower the shell under the oil. You're framing the taco shape here, however you would prefer not to un-puff the sides, on the off chance that you can help it.

12) Utilizing one tong, keep the taco squeezed under the oil. Utilizing the other, keep the top piece of the taco in any event two inches separated.

13) Eliminate when brilliant earthy colored to a paper towel. Rehash with the other 11 shells.

14) Stuff with taco meat and the entirety of your number one trimming!

Smoked Caramelized Onion Dip:

My hand crafted Smoked Caramelized Onion Dip requires ZERO bundles of anything, and is one of my #1 plunges to make for a group! Traeger caramelized onions AND garlic go into this, and you'll be scrambling for things to plunge!

Onion Dip Shopping List

1) 2 huge Vidalia or Walla sweet onions
2) 2 cloves garlic
3) sharp cream
4) cream cheddar
5) onion powder
6) s&p

12 ounces sharp cream

1) 4 ounces cream cheddar, room temperature
2) 1 cup smoked caramelized onions
3) 1 teaspoon smoked broiled garlic
4) 1/2 teaspoon salt
5) 1/4 teaspoon onion powder
6) run pepper

Method:

1) Take the entirety of the fixings and combine them until all around consolidated.
2) Spot in the refrigerator and chill for 3-4 hours before servings.

South Beach Diet Simple Pizza Sauce Recipe:

Ingredients:

1) One tablespoon tomato glue
2) 1 cup tomato puree
3) 1/8 teaspoon squashed red pepper pieces
4) Two teaspoons dried oregano
5) Two teaspoons dried basil
6) Two teaspoons dried thyme Directions:

Consolidate all in little pot and cook over low warmth for 15 minutes, or until sauce thickens.

Put starting five ingredients in a container. A tiny bit at a timed race in milk until no bunches remain. Warmth and blend until foaming and thickened. Blend in margarine until disintegrated. Spread on pizza outside layer; top with most adored embellishments. Unbelievable with grilled chicken strips on top!

A-1-DERFUL Mini Pizzas Recipe:

Ingredients:

1) 3/4-pound ground burger 1/4 cup minced onion
2) One can (6 oz. size) tomato stick three tablespoons A.1. Steak sauce
3) One teaspoon Italian herb seasonings 6 English bread rolls, split and toasted 2 cups cut mozzarella cheddar ground parmesan cheddar
4) 1/4 cup cut green onion Directions:

In tranquilize. Skillet, cook and break down meat until not, now pink; channel. Incorporate the onion and cook until sensitive. Mix in tomato stick, steak sauce, and Italian herb seasoning; cook until mix stews.

Spread bread leaves behind the meat mix. Top with cheeses and green onion. Spot on getting ready sheets. Singe 2 to 4 minutes or until cheddar is mollified.

Alsatian Bacon and Fresh Cheese Tart Recipe

Ingredients:

1) 1 group dynamic dry yeast
2) 1/2 cup warm water
3) 4 cups bread flour, notwithstanding flour for cleaning 1/2 cup cold water
4) One tablespoon genuine salt oil, for the bowl
5) 1/4-pound piece bacon cubed one tablespoon olive oil
6) 1/2 cup gently cut yellow onions
7) Three tablespoons yellow cornmeal, for cleaning compartment one enormous egg
8) One tablespoon, for the most part, helpful flour 1/4 cup ground Gruyere cheddar two

tablespoons water
9) 3/4 cup whole milk ricotta cheddar three tablespoons plain yogurt
10) press salt

Method:

The flammkuchen, or "blasting tart," is the Alsatian adjustment of pizza. All through the area, you'll find commonplace bistros that make a distinguishing strength of the dish. The floppy tarts are brought out from the wood-expending grill on a wooden strip, slid clearly onto the table, and ate up while they are about too hot to manage.

In a gigantic mixing bowl, join yeast and the warm water Let speak to 5 minutes Add the infection water and salt Begin including bread flour 1 cup immediately, blending incredible after each choice When player ends up being too firm to even think about evening consider mixing, move to a delicately floured surface and handle until smooth and reflexive (7 to 10 minutes) Place in a gently oiled bowl and go to cover blend with oil Cover and let climb until increased in mass, around 1 3/4 hours In a medium skillet over moderate warmth, render bacon in olive oil until bacon fat is melted and bacon is caramelized Transfer bacon to a plate with opened spoon and add onion to skillet Sauté until insignificantly mellowed (around 5 minutes) Cool to room temperature Preheat grill to 425 F Dust a pizza stone or significant warming sheet with cornmeal Whisk together Fromage Blanc, egg, and the 1 Tbsp flour Punch down blend and crease into as tremendous a circle or square shape as will fit on the warming sheet Transfer to orchestrated getting ready sheet Spread with Fromage Blanc mix to inside 3/4 inch of edge Top with onions and rendered bacon and sprinkle with ground cheddar Brush edge of blend with the 2 Tbsp water Bake until splendid dim hued (15 to 20 minutes)

Artichoke Turkey Pizza Recipe:

Ingredients:

1) 1 arranged thin Italian pizza outside layer (12-inch size)
2) 1 1/2 cup crushed Mozzarella cheddar
3) One can (14.5-ounce size) diced tomatoes with basil, garlic, and oregano, drained
4) 1 cup severed cooked turkey
5) One can (14-ounce size) artichoke hearts, drained, coarsely cut
6) One can (2.25-ounce size) cut dull olives, exhausted
7) 1/2 cup crushed Parmesan cheddar

Method:

Preheat oven to 450 degrees F. Spot outside layer on ungreased warming sheet. Sprinkle with mozzarella cheddar. Top with tomatoes, turkey, artichokes, olives, and Parmesan cheddar. Warmth 10 minutes, or until cheddar is condensed. In a medium significant skillet cook prosciutto and onion in oil over moderate warmth, mixing, until onion is loose. Oust skillet from the warmth and blend in arugula and salt and pepper to taste. Brains flour tortillas on two warming sheets and top with arugula mix and Parmesan. Warmth pizzas on upper and lower racks of oven, trading spots of getting ready sheets almost through warming, until edges are splendid, around 10 minutes.

Bacon Cheeseburger Upside-Down Pizza
Yield

Ingredients:

1) 1-pound lean ground meat
2) One medium onion, quartered, cut
3) One medium ring pepper, chop into diminished down strips six cuts bacon, crisp-cooked and deteriorated
4) 1 (14 1/2 ounce) can thick pizza sauce 3 Italian plum tomatoes
5) Six cuts cheddar

Method:

Warmth grill to 400 degrees F.
In a large pot, a dull shaded ground burger with onion and ringer pepper; channel. Blend in 6 cuts broke down bacon and pizza sauce. Spoon into ungreased 13 x 9-inch getting ready to dish. Sprinkle consistently with tomatoes; top with cheddar cuts.

Beating two eggs

1 cup milk

One tablespoon oil

1   cup all-around convenient flour 1/4 teaspoon salt

Two   slices bacon, crisp-cooked and broke down

In a medium bowl, beat eggs insignificantly. Incorporate milk and oil; mix well. Carefully spoon flour into evaluating cup; level off. Incorporate flour and salt; beat 2 minutes at medium speed. Pour consistently over cheddar cuts. Sprinkle with broke down bacon. Warmth at 400 degrees F for 20 to 30 minutes or until fixing is somewhat puffed and significant splendid darker.

* 1/2-pound ground meat
* 1 little onion, hacked
* 1 pre-arranged Italian bread chill outside layer
* 8 ounces would pizza have the option to the sauce
* 6 bacon strips, cooked and crumbled
* 20 dill pickle coin cuts
* 2 cups devastated mozzarella cheddar
* 2 cups devastated cheddar
* 1 teaspoon pizza or Italian seasonings

In a skillet, cook cheeseburger and onion until meat isn't, now pink and channel by then put in a protected spot. Spot covering on an ungreased 12-inch pizza dish. Spread sauce, top with burger mix, bacon, pickles and cheeses; sprinkle with seasonings. Warmth at 450 for 10 minutes or until cheeses have mellowed. Cut into cuts and serve.

Bacon Onion and Tomato Pizza Recipe:

Ingredients:

1) One tablespoon olive oil
2) One tablespoon oil for brushing on pitas
3) 2 cups cut onions
4) Salt and pepper to taste
5) Three tablespoons darker sugar
6) 4 Greek-style pita pieces of bread (at any rate six sneaks in separation over)
7) Garlic powder to taste
8) 1/2 cup mozzarella cheddar
9) Two gigantic tomatoes washed, cut 1/4-inch-thick, split at whatever point needed
10) 1 1/2 cup cut fresh spinach, optional
11) 8 cups cooked bacon, each chop down the center, secluded
12) One cup most cherished wrecked sharp upgraded cheddar.

Directions:

Preheat the oven to 400 degrees. Incorporate the cut onions and season with salt and pepper. Sauté the onions until fragile, around 3 to 5 minutes. Sprinkle with the dark shaded sugar and continue cooking until the onions turn a splendid darker.

Remove from the glow and put it in a sheltered spot. Recognize the pita bread on a getting ready sheet and brush each with a thin covering of olive oil. Sprinkle each with the garlic powder and subsequently around two tablespoons of the mozzarella cheddar. Top with a touch of the onions and a short time later coordinate the tomato cuts on the pita. At whatever point needed, beautify with a bit of the spinach in the canter. Sort out four bacon cuts on top. Warmth around 8 to 10 minutes or until the tomatoes begin to smooth. Oust from the stove and sprinkle each with 1/4 cup of the cheddar. Return to the oven and warmth until the cheddar disintegrates. Oust from the grill and serve.

Bacon Spinach Pizza Recipe:

Ingredients:

*   1 can (10-oz. size) Refrigerated Pizza Crust
*   1 pack (9-oz. size) Chopped Frozen Spinach
*   1 tablespoon oil
*   1/2 cup coarsely severed onion
*   1 pack (6-oz. size) refrigerated cooked Italian-style chicken chest strips, divided
*   2 cups crushed mozzarella cheddar
*   1 pack (2.8 to 3-oz. size) precooked bacon cuts, cut into 1/2-INCH pieces

Method:

Warmth oven to 400°F. Oil 15X10X1-INCH warming holder. Unroll hitter; place in the lobed holder. Starting at canter, press out hitter to edge of skillet. Get ready at 400°F. for 9 to 13 minutes or until edges are light splendid dull shaded.

Meanwhile, cook spinach as facilitated in the group. Channel well; press to oust liquid. Warmth oil in a little skillet over medium-high warmth until hot. Incorporate onion; cook and blend 3 to 4 minutes or until fragile, mixing intermittently. Oust somewhat arranged structure from the grill. Top body with spinach, onion, chicken, cheddar, and bacon. Return to stove; set up an additional 9 to 12 minutes or until cheddar is broken down. Cut into squares.

Arranged Pizza Sandwich Recipe:

Ingredients:

*   1-pound Lean Ground Beef
*   15 ounces Tomato Sauce
*   15 ounces Pizza Sauce
*   1 teaspoon Oregano Leaves
*   2 cups Biscuit Baking Mix

*   1 Egg; Lg.
*   2/3 cup Milk
*   8 ounces Cheese
*   2 ounces Mushrooms
*   1/4 cup Parmesan Cheese; Grated Directions:
* Use one 8-oz heap of cut strategy American or mozzarella cheddar.

Method:

Warmth the stove to 400 degrees F. Cook and blend the meat in a large skillet until dull hued. Direct off the wealth fat. Blend in half of the tomato sauce, and the oregano leaves into the meat mix. Warmth to rising by then decline the glow and stew, uncovered, for 10 minutes. While the meat mix is stewing, mix the planning mix, egg, and milk. Measure out 3/4 cup of the player and put it in a sheltered spot. Spread the remainder of the hitter in a lobed, getting ready compartment 9 X 9 X 2-INCHES. Spreading similarly. Layer 4 cups of the cheddar, the meat mix, the mushrooms, and the remainder of the cheddar on the tomato sauce. Spoon the held player on the most noteworthy purpose of the cheddar. Sprinkle the player top with the ground Parmesan cheddar and plan, uncovered until it is splendid dull shaded, 20 to 25 minutes. Cool for 5 minutes before cutting into squares and serving.

Cheeseburger Tortilla Pizza Recipe

Ingredients:

*   1-pound lean ground cheeseburger
*   1 medium onion - cut
*   1 teaspoon dried oregano leaves
*   1 teaspoon salt
*   4 tremendous (10 inch) flour tortillas
*   1 medium tomato - seeded and cut
*   1 tablespoon fresh basil leaves - gently cut
*   1 cup Mozzarella cheddar - devastated
*   1/4 cup Parmesan cheddar - ground

Methods:

Warmth grill to 400ºF. Dull shaded ground cheeseburger and onion in a skillet over medium warmth 8 to 10 minutes or until meat isn't, now pink. Pour off drippings. Blend oregano and salt into the meat.

Delicately brush tortillas with oil. Plan tortillas on two huge warming sheets in 400ºF oven for 3 minutes. Spoon cheeseburger mix consistently over top of each tortilla; top with a comparable proportion of tomato. Sprinkle with basil and cheeses. Return to grill and warmth 12 to 14 minutes or until tortillas are gently sung.

Breakfast Pizza Recipe:

Ingredients:

* 1/2-pound hotdog, cooked and depleted
* 1 bundle Crescent rolls
* 5 eggs
* 1/4 teaspoon dry mustard
* 1/4 teaspoon pepper
* 1/4 cup milk
* 1 cup hash tans
* 1 cup ground cheddar

Methods:

Preheat stove to 375F. Oil an 8"x8" or 9"x9" container. Unfurl Crescent folds into strips and press together on base and sides. Whisk eggs, milk, mustard, and pepper. Sprinkle the frankfurter and potatoes, at that point the cheddar on Crescent rolls. Pour egg blend overall. Sprinkle with Parmesan cheddar. Prepare 40-45 minutes until no fluid in focus.

Broccoli Turkey Pizza Recipe

Ingredients:

*   1/3 cup low fat mayonnaise
*   1 tablespoon Dionisio mustard
*   1/2 teaspoon pepper
*   2 1/2 cups cleaved crisp or defrosted solidified broccoli
*   2 cups cubed cooked turkey
*   1 cup destroyed cheddar
*   1 (12-inch size) round Boboli or other covering

Method:

In a medium bowl, consolidate mayonnaise, Dionisio, and pepper. Mix in broccoli, turkey, and cheddar. Spread turkey blend on the outside layer and prepare at 425F for 12 minutes or until gently seared.

Air pocket Pizza Recipe:

Ingredients:

*   1 1/2-pound meat, caramelized and depleted
*   15 ounces pizza sauce
*   1 can refrigerated buttermilk scones
*   12 ounces destroyed pizza mix cheddar

Bearings:

Add pizza sauce to ground meat. Cut bread rolls in quarters and spot in a lobed 9X13 dish. Top with hamburger blend. Prepare at 400F degrees for 20 minutes. Sprinkle with cheddar and prepare until cheddar liquefies. Let stand 5-10 minutes before serving. You can include your preferred garnishes alongside the meat before heating.

* three bundles (7.5-ounce size) buttermilk rolls

* 1 container (14-ounce size) spaghetti sauce

* 3 cups mozzarella cheddar, separated

* 1 colossal clove garlic, slashed fine

Preheat stove to 350 degrees. Quarter bread rolls utilizing kitchen shears and spot in a medium-sized bowl. Mix in 1 cup of sauce, 2 cups of cheddar, and the garlic. Include whatever fixings you like and blend to consolidate. Spread blend in a lobed 9-by-13 container. Pour remaining sauce and cheddar over the top. Prepare for 30-35 minutes.

Butternut Squash, Bacon, And Rosemary Pizza Recipe:

Ingredients:

* 1 1/2-pound butternut squash
* 1 tablespoon vegetable oil
* 1/2 cup water
* 6 tablespoons unsalted margarine, liquefied and kept warm
* ten sheets phyllo stacked between sheets of wax paper and secured with a kitchen towel
* 9 tablespoons parmesan cheddar - crisply ground
* 6 cuts bacon cut into 1/2-INCH pieces, cooked until fresh, and depleted
* 1 tablespoon crisp rosemary leaves - minced
* 6 scallion greens - slashed
* 1 little red onion cut flimsy and isolated into pieces Directions:

Method:

Quarter squash the long way and dispose of seeds. Strip squash cautiously and cut into 3/4-inch pieces. In a sizeable overwhelming skillet cook squash in oil over moderate warmth, mixing every so often, 2 minutes.

Add water and salt to taste and stew, secured, until squash is merely delicate, around 10 minutes. Stew squash, revealed until practically all water is vanished, around 5 minutes. In a nourishment processor, purée squash with salt and pepper to taste. Squash purée might be made one day ahead and chilled, secured. Preheat grill to 400°F. Softly brush an enormous preparing sheet with some spread and put one sheet phyllo on margarine. Gently brush phyllo with some outstanding spread and sprinkle with one tablespoon Parmesan. Put another sheet of phyllo over cheddar, squeezing it immovably with the goal that it clings to the base layer. Spread, sprinkle with cheddar, and layer remaining phyllo in a similar way, finishing with a sheet of phyllo. Delicately brush top sheet with outstanding margarine. Overlap in all sides 1/4 inch, squeezing to top sheet, and overlay up a 1/4-inch fringe, pleating corners. Spread squash purée uniformly on phyllo outside layer and top with bacon, rosemary, scallion greens, and onion. Heat pizza in the canter of the appliance until the outside layer is brilliant, around 15 minutes.

Camper's Pizza Recipe:

Ingredients:

* 12 ounces ground hamburger - 80% lean

* 1 medium onion - cleaved

* 1/2 teaspoon salt

* 8 ounces refrigerated bow rolls

* 8 ounces pizza sauce

* 4 ounces mushroom stems and pieces - depleted and slashed

* 2 1/4 ounces ready olives - hollowed and cut

* 1/3 cup green chime pepper - coarsely hacked

* 4 ounces destroyed Mozzarella cheddar

* 1 teaspoon dried oregano leaves - squashed

Method:

Cook ground meat and onion in all around prepared 11 to 12-INCH overwhelming skillet with heat-verification handle over medium coals* until not, at this point pink, mixing periodically to separate hamburger. Expel hamburger blend to paper towel; season with salt. Pour off drippings, leaving skillet "lobed." Separate bow moves mixture triangles; place in skillet, squeezing edges together to frame base outside layer and 1-inch edge up the side of skillet. A spread portion of pizza sauce over batter; spoon ground hamburger blend over the sauce.

Top with mushrooms, olives, and ringer pepper. Pour remaining sauce over all; sprinkle with cheddar and oregano. Spot skillet in the focus of lattice over medium coals.

Canadian Bacon Pizza Recipe

Ingredients:

*   1 (12 inch) pizza covering - unbaked

*   1 cup pizza sauce

* 2/3 cup destroyed mozzarella cheddar

* 6 ounces Canadian bacon - cut in bits

* 1/2 cup meagrely cut crisp mushrooms

* 1 little green or red ringer pepper - cut in rings

* 1/2 teaspoon squashed dried oregano

* 1/2 teaspoon squashed dried basil

* crushed red pepper drops

Method:

Preheat grill to 450F. Spot the unbaked pizza covering on an ungreased non-stick pizza dish. Spread the pizza sauce over the outside layer, leaving a 1-inch fringe around the edge. Sprinkle with half of the cheddar. Orchestrate the Canadian bacon on the cheddar, covering uniformly. Top with mushroom cuts and chime pepper rings.

Sprinkle equitably with oregano, basil, and red pepper pieces. Top with outstanding cheddar. Heat for 13 to 15 minutes, until the outside layer is fresh and the cheddar is dissolved and seared.

Bacon Pizza Recipe:

Ingredients:

*   2 tablespoons margarine

*   2 medium pears, cored, each cut into 12 the long way cuts

*   2 tablespoons solidly pressed dark colored sugar

*   4 singular pizza outside layers (8 inches)

*   1/2 cup alfredo sauce

*   1 cup destroyed mozzarella cheddar

*   3/4 cup disintegrated blue cheddar

*   3/4 cup bacon bits (genuine)

Method:

Liquefy spread in medium skillet on medium warmth. Include pears; sprinkle uniformly with dark-colored sugar. Cook 2 to 3 minutes or until sugar is softened, and pears are equally covered, mixing every so often. Expel skillet from heat; put in a safe spot Spread every pizza outside layer with 2 Tbsp. Alfredo sauce; top each with layers of 1/4 cup of the mozzarella cheddar, 3 Tbsp. of the blue cheddar, 3 Tbsp. of the bacon, and six pear cuts. Spot on the heating sheet. Heat at 425 F for 6 to 8 minutes or until garnish is brilliant and bubbly.

Pancetta Pizza Recipe:

Ingredients:

* 1 cup warm water (105 degrees)

* 1 1/4-ounce bundle yeast

* 3 cups generally useful flour

* 1 teaspoon salt

* 1 teaspoon sugar

* 2 tablespoons olive oil

* 2 onions

* 2 teaspoons olive oil

* 1 1/2 teaspoon salt

* 1 1/2 cup coarsely ground fontina

* 6 cuts pancetta, cooked until fresh

* 1 clove garlic, cut down the middle

* 1 shower of olive oil

* salt and pepper to taste

Method:

Empty the water into a large bowl. Sprinkle in the yeast and sugar and mix to break down. Let it remain until the blend starts to bubble. This should take around 5 minutes. Begin it once again with another bundle of yeast.

Mix in 1 cup of flour, the salt, and one tablespoon olive oil. Blend in with a wooden spoon until altogether consolidated. Include the rest of the flour 1/2 cup at once, blending after every expansion.

On a daintily floured surface, manipulate mixture until smooth and versatile, around 10 minutes. Oil an enormous bowl with the staying olive oil. Spot batter in an oiled bowl spread with saran wrap and a warm drying towel, and let the mixture ascend in a warm spot until multiplied in mass. This will take 1 to 1/2 hours.

Punch down the mixture and return it to the floured surface. Gap mixture into two balls and spread each with cling wrap, leaving space for development. Permit to twofold in size once more. Caramelized Onions: Heat oil in enormous non-stick salute containers over medium warmth. Include meagrely cut onions and season with salt; saute 5 minutes. Diminish warmth to medium-low. Mix now and again to get a smooth shading. Cook until extremely delicate and a rich, brilliant shading creates, around 20 minutes longer. Cool somewhat. Preheat grill to 475 degrees. Turn out two batter circles on a softly floured surface to 8-inch adjusts. Sprinkle two heating sheets or pizza stones with cornmeal. Rub a liberal shower of olive oil on the batter. Rub raw garlic clove all over the mixture. Top with fontina, caramelized onions, and pancetta. Season with salt and pepper. Heat pizza for 10-12 minutes, until foaming and fresh.

Cheddar Steak Pizza Recipe:

Ingredients:

*   1 arranged pizza outside (12 inches)

*   1/2 cup grill sauce or pizza sauce

*   1 bundle (6 oz.) Grilled Beef Steak Strips

*   2 cups Shredded Cheese

*   Sliced green pepper and onion

Method:

Spread pizza outside with grill sauce. Top with meat steak strips, cheddar, green pepper, and onion. Spot on the treated sheet. Heat at 450 F for 8 to 10 minutes or until cheddar is liquefied.

*   1 (10 oz. size) slight pre-prepared pizza shell

*   4 ounces cream cheddar, mellowed

*   3/4 teaspoon Italian flavoring

*   1/4 teaspoon crisply ground pepper

*   2 cups destroyed leaf lettuce

*   1 cup finely destroyed Co-Jack cheddar

* 3/4 cup cleaved new tomato

* 7 cuts bacon, cooked until fresh, cleaved

* olives, cut (discretionary) Directions:

Preheat grill to 400 degrees. Spot pizza shell on the prepared sheet. Warmth in grill 5 minutes or until somewhat fresh. Expel from the stove and let cool marginally. Join cream cheddar, Italian flavoring, and pepper. Spread on pizza shell to inside 1/2 inch of edge. Sprinkle with lettuce, Co-Jack cheddar, tomato, and bacon. Top with sliced olives whenever wanted. Cut pizza into wedges and serve.

Mushy Jalapeno and Egg Pizza Recipe:

Ingredients:

* 6 eggs

* 6 cups destroyed cheddar

* 6 cups destroyed mozzarella cheddar

* 6 ounces cut jalapenos

* Pepperoni, cut

Method:

Blend eggs, cheddar, and jalapenos. Fill rectangular goulash. Lay cuts of pepperoni on top and spot into 350-degree F stove. Cook until cheddar is brilliant (around 10-15 minutes). Let represent 5 minutes, cut into 2-INch squares, and serve.

Preheated stove to 475. Blend the above ingredients for 10 minutes in a robust blender or manipulate by hand. Presently include 2 1/2 cups of flour. Blend for 15 minutes in a robust blender with a battered snare or by hand. Presently the mixture must ascent. The batter ought to be in a massive bowl in a warm spot, secured with a drying towel.
If it isn't warm in the kitchen, turn the stove on to the least setting (close to 100) and let the mixture ascend in the bowl in the appliance, secured by the towel. Let ascend just because (about 60 minutes) and punch down the batter. Let rise once more, punch down, and use. Push the battery out level with your fingers, in a high-sided pizza container, or a sizeable dark iron skillet. Spread with mozzarella cheddar. Spread with tomato sauce with Italian herbs and flavors included. Spread with hacked garlic, green peppers, cut pepperoni, sweet Italian sausage, cut mushrooms, cleaned onions, or whatever to taste. Sprinkle with ground Romano or Parmesan cheddar. Cook in a grill at 475 until done, around 15 to 20 minutes relying upon garnishes and thickness of the outside layer and how fresh you need it cooked.

Ciro's Pizza Recipe:

Ingredients:

*   1/2-pound flour

*   1/2-ounce pastry specialists' yeast

*   1 tablespoon water to mix yeast

*   1 tablespoon olive oil, in addition to extra to hose pizza at the end

*   Salt and pepper

*   1 egg

*   1/4 cup high temp water

*   2 jars (1 pound 12-OUNCE) crisp egg-molded tomatoes, cleaned, seeded and generally slashed

*   2 teaspoons escapades

*   1/2 little tin anchovies in oil, depleted

*   5 cuts mozzarella cheddar

*   ten dark olive pants

*   1 sprig oregano

*   1 little garlic clove, finely cut

*   Freshly ground dark pepper, for decorating

Method:

Spot the flour in a bowl. Make a well in the inside, add the yeast blended to glue with water, and afterward the olive oil, salt, pepper, and egg. Combine and afterward slim glue with boiling water until it looks like biting gum and leaves from the hands. Manipulate for around 3 minutes until it no longer sticks to hands. Shape batter into a ball spread with a bowl and permit to stand 30 minutes. Massage again and afterward get the mixture and haul it out with the fingers, turning it around. Oil a heating sheet and preheat broiler to 500 degrees F. Spot the batter onto the heating sheet, spreading it out to frame 12-inch breadth round shape. The edge ought to be somewhat thicker than the middle. Enhancement with tomatoes, escapades, anchovies, mozzarella cheddar, dark olive parts, oregano leaves, garlic, and pepper. Sprinkle with oil and spot into the stove for 20 minutes. Spot on serving dish.

Club Pizza Recipe:

Ingredients:

*   1 prebaked slim Italian pizza outside layer

*   10 ounces arranged Alfredo sauce

*   10 ounces hacked solidified spinach - defrosted and depleted

*   1 cup cubed cooked chicken

*   1 cup hacked tomato

*   6 cuts bacon - cooked and disintegrated

Method:

Warmth stove to 450F degrees. Spot pizza outside layer in a large ungreased treat sheet. Spread hull with Alfredo sauce. Top with spinach, chicken, tomato, and bacon. Prepare at 450F degrees for 8 to 10 minutes or until thoroughly warmed.

In a little bowl, consolidate cream cheddar, mayonnaise, and horseradish sauce and mix well. Spread over the pizza covering. Top with ham, plum tomatoes, and lettuce and sprinkle with a plate of mixed greens dressing. Cut into wedges and serve right away.

Corncake Pizza Wheels Recipe:

Ingredients:

*   1-pound ground meat

*   1 can (16-ounce size) kidney beans, washed and depleted

*   1 can (8-ounce size) tomato sauce

*   4 teaspoons bean stew powder

*   1 container (4-ounce size) diced pimientos, depleted

*   1 can (4-ounce size) cleaved green chilies, depleted

*   1 cup destroyed cheddar

*   2 tablespoons cornmeal

*   2 tubes (11-1/2-ounce size) refrigerated corncake turns

*   Shredded lettuce, cut tomatoes, and acrid cream

Method:

In a skillet, cook the hamburger over medium warmth until not, at this point, pink; channel. Include the beans, tomato sauce, and stew powder. Stew revealed until the liquid has dissipated. Expel from the warmth and cold. Mix in the pimientos, chilies, and cheddar; put in a safe spot. Sprinkle two-lobed 14-IN. Pizza dish with corn-dinner. Pat the hoecake batter into a 14-IN. Hover on each dish. With a blade, cut a 7-in. X in the canter of the batter. Cut another 7-in. X to frame eight pie-formed wedges in the middle. Spoon the filling around the edge of the mixture. Overlay purposes of batter over filling; fold under the ring and squeeze to seal (filling will be noticeable). Heat at 400F for 15-20 minutes or until brilliant dark-colored. Fill focus with lettuce, tomatoes, and harsh cream.

Corn Tortilla Pizzas Recipe

Ingredients:

* 1 1/4-pound ground burger

* 1 little onion, sliced

* 1/2 cup sliced green pepper

* 3 containers (6-ounce size) tomato stick

* 1 1/4 cup water

* 1 cup salsa

* 2 cups fresh or hardened corn

* 1 1/2 cup cut new tomatoes

* 3/4 cup cut prepared olives

* 1 envelope taco enhancing

* 3 teaspoons garlic powder

* 1 1/2 teaspoon dried parsley drops

* 1/2 teaspoon dried oregano

* 1/8 teaspoon salt

* 1/4 teaspoon pepper

* 32 corn or flour tortillas (6-inch size)

* 8 cups obliterated mozzarella cheddar

Method:

In a skillet, cook cheeseburger, onion, and green pepper over medication. Heat until meat isn't, now pink; channel. In a bowl, merge tomato pastes and water until blended; incorporate salsa. Blend into meat corn, tomatoes, olives, and seasonings. Spot tortillas on ungreased warming sheets. Spread each with 1/4 cup meat mix to inside 1/2 inch of edge and sprinkle with 1/4 cup of cheddar. Warmth at 375F for 5-7 minutes or until mellowed.

Crazy Crust Pizza Recipe:

Ingredients:

*   1 cup flour

*   1 teaspoon salt

*   1 teaspoon Italian seasoning or oregano

*   1/8 teaspoon pepper

*   2 eggs

*   2/3 cup milk Topping

*   1-pound ground burger/sausage

* 1 cup pepperoni

* 1/4 cup sliced onion

* 1 cup pizza sauce

* 8 ounces tomato sauce mixed in with oregano and pepper

* 1 cup wrecked Mozzarella cheddar

* 1 can (4 oz.) mushrooms Directions:

Method:

In medium skillet darker ground meat, seasoning to taste. (No convincing motivation to darker pepperoni). Channel well, put in a sheltered spot. Tenderly oil and build-up 12- or 14-inch pizza skillet or 10X15 jam move dish with flour or corn supper. Plan hitter by mixing to flour, salt, Italian enhancing, pepper, eggs, and milk in a touch of mixing bowl. Pour hitter in skillet, tilting dish, so player covers the base. Compose fixing of meat and onions over the player. Warmth on-base rack in a 425-degree oven for 20-25 minutes or until pizza is significant splendid dim shaded. Oust from stove; shower with pizza sauce and sprinkle with cheddar. Top with mushrooms or various toppings. Return to the stove for 10-15 minutes until cheddar is melted and sauce is bubbly.

Crazy Crust Pizza II Recipe

Ingredients:

* 1 cup flour

* 3 eggs

* 2/3 cup milk

* 1/2-pound ground meat

* 1/2 cup onions

* Pizza sauce

* Cheese

* Pepperoni

* Mushrooms

* Bell pepper

* Onions

Method:

Mix flour, eggs, and milk. Beat 2 to 3 minutes. Dull shaded ground cheeseburger and onions. Oil getting ready sheet; pour flour mix onto the sheet. Incorporate meat and onions. Warmth for 25 minutes at 425 degrees F. Remove from grill. Incorporate sauce, cheddar, and remaining ingredients. Set up an additional 10 minutes.

Dull shaded meat and pepper together and channel oil. Prepare a player and fill a lubed pizza dish. Tilt holder, so the player covers the base. Genius meat mix, onion, and mushrooms over the hitter.

Get ready at 425 for 20 minutes or until splendid darker. Oust from the stove and incorporate pizza sauce and cheddar. Return to the stove for ten extra minutes or until cheddar mellow. Detect a square of foil on a treat sheet. Put the burger mix on the foil. Pat out the meat entirely into a 10-inch float around 1/2 inch thick. Build up a standing edge around 1-inch high all around the edge of the circle. This makes a meat "frame" for your pizza (make sure to make the meat edge adequately high and firm enough so it will thwart the meat crushes and soup sauce from ascending). Spread the rest of the ten 3/4-ounce container of tomato soup over meat. Top cheeseburger outside layer with Mozzarella cheddar and more oregano and mushrooms. Warmth at 450 degrees for 15 minutes or until done.

Straightforward Bake Oven Deep Dish Pizza Recipe

Ingredients:

*   2 tablespoons for the most part valuable flour

*   1/8 teaspoon getting the ready powder

*   Dash of salt

*   1 teaspoon margarine

*   2 1/4 teaspoons milk

*   1 tablespoon pizza sauce

*   1 1/2 tablespoon demolished mozzarella cheddar Directions:

Method:

Combine flour, getting ready powder, salt and margarine until blend seems like medium-sized pieces. Bit by bit incorporate milk while blending. Shape hitter into a ball and spot into a lobed compartment. Use your fingers to pat the blend similarly over the base of the holder, by then up the sides. Pour the sauce similarly over the hitter by then sprinkle with the cheddar. Get ready 20 mins. Oust. Make the French Bread blend recipe on any occasion one day as of now in case you can. Transform the blend out into the condition of a pizza, put it on a pizza dish, and put it in a sheltered spot. It will keep in the more relaxed present moment. Set up the dried mushrooms as showed by conveyed plans (douse, wash, cut, resoak, wash, channel). If the snails are unnecessarily enormous (more significant than a garlic clove), then cut them in pieces. Channel the snails well. Mellow the spread in a warming dish, incorporate the snails, squashed garlic, around 1/2 salt, and ground dull pepper to taste.

Put the bread-hitter compartment on the top rack of the stove and the snails on the base rack of the oven, and cook them both for 10 minutes. Take them out. Spread the tomato sauce in an even layer on the bread, by then sprinkle the Raclette cheddar over it. Incorporate the snails, and a while later, the mushrooms. Sprinkle with new parmesan cheddar, salt, and pepper. Get ready at 425 degrees F. in the top rack for 12 minutes (base rack will devour the frame). Get it, use fondue cheddar or a Gruyere.

Fig and Prosciutto Pizza Recipe:

Ingredients:

*   1 group dynamic dry yeast, that has reliably been in a cooler

*   1 contact of sugar

*   3/4 cup warm water, not any more sizzling than 110 (from the tap)

*   3 cups commonly helpful flour

*   2 tablespoons olive oil

*   2 teaspoons sea salt

*   Olive oil for the resting bowl Pizza

*   1 half quart new figs, stems ousted, slice to the thickness of a pea.

*   1/2-pound Prosciutto di Parma from San Daniele.

*   1 tablespoon fennel seeds

*   Extra virgin olive oil

*   pizza player

Method:

For Pizza Dough: "Start" the yeast by mixing it in with the sugar and water for around seven to ten minutes. Put the yeast, sugar and water mix in your remarkable blender, fitted with the blend catch. Incorporate the flour, olive oil, and salt. Start the machine and let mix until a blend ball structures. Stop the machine and let the hitter rest for three minutes. Heartbeat the machine on numerous occasions. Flour on the counter and put the blend on the floured surface. Handle for five minutes.

Coat a medium-sized bowl with some olive oil. Put the player in the bowl, by then turn the blend over, so the different sides are made sure about with a film of oil. Spread the bowl with cling wrap. 2 hours so the blend can rise. Following two hours, punch the hitter from the inside to level. Put it on a floured counter. Chop the player down the canter, and freeze one half for at some point later. Crease the other half into a ball and spread it with the bowl for thirty minutes.

For Fig and Prosciutto Pizza: Toast the fennel seeds in a hot, dry dish around five minutes. Put in a sheltered spot. Warmth your oven to 4750 with a pizza stone on the most raised rack. Use a treat sheet dish that has no edges. Spread it well with Wonda flour or cornmeal. Uncover the blend to the size of the pizza stone.

Move the blend onto the floured sheet dish. Spread out a layer of prosciutto, by then the figs, on the blend. Sprinkle the pizza with the toasted fennel. Move the pizza to the pizza stone by putting the sheet compartment on the stone and quickly pulling the plate away, so the pizza slides.

Warmth for five minutes or until the base of the outside is splendid darker. Oust the pizza from the stone by using the sheet dish and a significant spatula. Not sometime before serving, put the pizza onto a cutting load up. Shower it well with the extra virgin olive oil and cut it into squares.

Pellet Grill Beef Birria Tacos:

Our Pellet Grill Beef Birria Tacos formula may be a significant piece to SAY, yet you will go insane for this delicate meal beef that has been smoked and braised in a natively constructed stew sauce prior to getting destroyed, stuffed into tortillas that are canvassed in the consommé, lastly seared on your level top iron until they are fresh.

Beef Birria Shopping List

1) 4-ish pounds of beef broil
2) adobo preparing mix
3) 8 red Anaheim or bring forth stew peppers
4) Bring forth stew powder
5) chipotle peppers in adobo
6) corn tortillas
7) onion
8) cilantro
9) cheddar

Step by step instructions to cook beef birria

1) When the beef is seared, throw it into a dispensable foil skillet and stick it on your smoker for 1/2 hours at 180-200°.

2) While it is cooking those initial two hours, broil your peppers that will in the end turn into your consommé.

3) Following 1/2 hours, turn the flame broil up to 300°. Allow the peppers to remain on the flame broil for an additional 30 minutes, checking at regular intervals and eliminating before they consume.

Fire up the frying pan

When the meat is finished cooking the time has come to start up your Blackstone. You'll need it on medium to medium-low warmth. You need your tacos to fresh up yet not consume.

Set up your entire circumstance in a mechanical production system. Broiling these goes quick, so you'll must have all you require in arm's range to complete it.

Plunge your tortillas in the consommé and spread them out on the iron. Top the WHOLE tortilla with cheddar, and afterward 50% of it with some beef, some cilantro, and some diced onions (on the off chance that you are into such a thing).

Overlap the shell over, press gently with the spatula, and fry on the two sides until the shell is fresh and the cheddar is dissolved.

1) 2 pounds beef throw shoulder broil
2) 2 pounds beef tri-tip broil, top round, base round, or another comparable beef cook
3) 4 tablespoons Adobo preparing mix
4) 1 teaspoon salt
5) 1 teaspoon garlic powder
6) 3 tablespoons canola oil
7) 8 huge, red, gentle chile peppers, (for example, Anaheim or red Hatch peppers)
8) 1 tablespoon beef bouillon
9) 1 teaspoon onion powder
10) 1 teaspoon garlic powder
11) 1 teaspoon salt
12) 1 tablespoon bean stew powder
13) 1 tablespoon incubate stew powder (discretionary)
14) 1 tablespoon oregano
15) 3 cloves garlic
16) 1 little onion, diced
17) 1/3 cup apple juice vinegar
18) 2 chipotle peppers in adobo sauce
19) 4 cups heated water

Earthy coloured and smoke the meat

1) Turn on your pellet flame broil to "smoke" at 180-200°.

2) 3D shapes your beef and season with the adobo, salt, and garlic powder. Earthy colored the meat on your level top frying pan in a touch of oil, or in a cast-iron skillet on the burner.

3) Put the sautéed 3D shapes of dish into a barbecue safe high-sided skillet or Dutch Oven, revealed.

4) Cut the peppers down the middle longwise and eliminate the seeds and the stem. Spot on the flame broil alongside the meat.

5) Smoke at 180-200° for 1/2 hours.

6) Turn the barbecue up to 300° and cook the peppers for an extra 30 minutes.

7) Make the consommé

8) Eliminate the peppers from the barbecue, place into a blender with the beef bouillon, onion powder, garlic powder, bean stew powder, oregano, garlic, onion, apple juice vinegar, chipotle peppers, and boiling water.

9) Mix until smooth, and dump over the beef lumps.

10) Braise the meat

11) Cover firmly and keep on cooking for another 2-4 hours, or until your beef is shred able and delicate. The occasions will shift dependent on your beef and your barbecue.

12) When the beef is delicate, eliminate it from the consommé and shred it with some utensils or two or three forks. Hold the consommé for some other time.

Fire up the level top

Preheat your Blackstone to medium warmth. Set out a little avocado oil and let it get hot.

While it is warming, plunge your flour tortillas in the consume and spot on the level top frying pan. Top the entire tortilla with cheddar, and half of it with a portion of the destroyed beef, onions, and cilantro.

Overlay over the unfilled portion of the tortilla and delicately push down. Cook for an extra 1-2 minutes, and flip. Keep cooking until the opposite side is fresh and afterward eliminate from the frying pan.

EAT!

Serve the tacos with any sort of fixing you like (I like lettuce and sharp cream with salsa) and a little dish of the consume for plunging.

Notes

On the off chance that you can't discover new peppers for cooking, you can substitute bean stew powder all things considered.

An assortment of bean stew powder is ideal. Models incorporate ancho, papilla, and guajillo. These assortments and others can be found in the Mexican zest part of your nearby food merchant.

Check your meal during the wet cooking stage to ensure the water doesn't vanish! In the event that you have the container covered firmly, it shouldn't, however it never damages straightening out something over the top.

THE TRAEGER GRILL BIBLE COOKBOOK 2021: THE ULTIMATE GUIDE.

365 Days of Delicious, Healthy & Tasty BBQ Recipes for Beginners & Advanced Pitmasters

AUTHOR
STEVEN JOHNSON

This document is geared towards providing exact and reliable information with regards to the topic and issue covered. The publication is sold with the idea that the publisher is not required to render accounting, officially permitted, or otherwise, qualified services. If advice is necessary, legal or professional, a practiced individual in the profession should be ordered.

From a Declaration of Principles which was accepted and approved equally by a Committee of the American Bar Association and a Committee of Publishers and Associations.

The information provided herein is stated to be truthful and consistent, in that any liability, in terms of inattention or otherwise, by any usage or abuse of any policies, processes, or directions contained within is the solitary and utter responsibility of the recipient reader. Under no circumstances will any legal responsibility or blame be held against the publisher for any reparation, damages, or monetary loss due to the information herein, either directly or indirectly.

Respective authors own all copyrights not held by the publisher.

The information herein is offered for informational purposes solely, and is universal as so. The presentation of the information is without contract or any type of guarantee assurance.

The trademarks that are used are without any consent, and the publication of the trademark is without permission or backing by the trademark owner. All trademarks and brands within this book are for clarifying purposes only and are owned by the owners themselves, not affiliated with this document.

WHAT IS TRAEGER WOOD PELLET GRILL?

A Traeger is a wood pellet grill. It uses proprietary wood pellets as fuel. This is different from a wood grill, and especially a charcoal grill.
Pellet grills are an exciting advancement in barbecuing. Most commonly known as "smokers," these grills are powered by hardwood pellets and act more like an outdoor oven than a standard gas or charcoal grill.

Wood pellet grills are one of the hottest trends in grilling right now. And Traeger is the top brand of pellet grill. If you just got one or are about to, you've no doubt wondered how to use a Traeger wood pellet grill.

Pellet grills use wood pellets as their fuel but also require an electrical outlet for power. They have 5 basic parts: the hopper, controller, the auger, the fire pot & the fan. They are much more accurate & simpler to operate than most grills. All new models even come with WIFI & can be controlled on a mobile device.

TRAEGER GRILL PELLETS BRIEF HISTORY

Joe Traeger is the inventor of the wood pellet grill. He came up with the idea after he noticed his gas grill was in flames as he was preparing to cook for his family.

That was in 1988. Today Traeger Grills has expanded to several different models of grills, from their Pro Series to their Timberline Series.

And Traeger has become the most well-known brand on the market. Pellet grills give consumers the flavor of wood smoke with the convenience of a gas grill.

Wood pellet grills use real wood, all-natural wood pellets as fuel. Unlike propane, natural gas, or charcoal grills, burning pellets is not harmful to the environment. They come in a variety of flavors and are FDA approved.

With several models of grills that boast 6-in-1 ability, it's no wonder they are so popular.

COMPONENTS OF TRAEGER WOOD PELLET GRILL

Pellet grills use wood pellets as their fuel but also require an electrical outlet for power.

They have 5 basic parts:
- The hopper
- The controller
- The auger
- The fire pot
- The fan.

They are much more accurate and simpler to operate than most grills. All new models even come with WIFI and can be controlled on a mobile device.

But how does a wood pellet grill work?
Pellet grills consist of five basic parts: the hopper, controller, the auger, the fire pot, and the fan. To start with, let's review each part, what it does, and how it works:

Controller

Wood pellet grills have the convenience of simple controls. Simply power on the grill and set it to whatever temperature you like. Just like you would your oven.
All current models of Tragers have this LCD style control panel.

If you see one with the old-school dial with temp settings marked on the grill, that is an older model. Nothing wrong with that, but they don't have all the modern advances that the new Traegers do, and if you see one in a store, it should definitely be discounted.

Hopper

The hopper is where you put the wood pellets.
They automatically feed down into the auger which moves them forward towards the firepot. You can open the hopper lid to check on pellet levels and add more at any time.
Traeger makes 13 different flavors of pellets. Their pellets are made from 100% natural, food-grade hardwood.

Auger

The auger is how the fire is fed.
The auger is located at the very bottom of the hopper. You just pour in the pellets into the hopper and gravity naturally forces them down into the auger which is rotating.
The auger moves the pellets from the hopper to the firepot. You can set it to move the pellets quickly if you want a hot, fast fire.
Set it to move the pellets gradually for low, slow cooking.

Firepot

The "HotRod" at the bottom of the fire pot ignites the wood pellets and creates the fire.

Fan

The fan stokes the fire. Variable speeds circulate the smoke and heat for even cooking.

To actually use your Traeger grill, just set the temperature just as you would an oven. The digital controller ensures consistent cooking temperatures while cooking.

Many models are even WiFi-enabled. This allows you to control your grill from anywhere using their app on your phone or smart home device.

That's it. Easy peasy.

Are you in the market for a new grill, but aren't sure if a Traeger is right for you?

Can you use a Traeger as a grill or just a smoker?

Absolutely. It can do both of those things and more!

Traeger boasts their grills are a "6-in-1" grill. All of their grills can:
- Grill
- Smoke
- Bake
- Roast
- Braise
- Barbeque

Because it heats using indirect heat, grilling is a bit slower than on a traditional grill.

Because it is an electric grill, it can't get as hot as a charcoal grill or even a propane grill. Trager grills get up to 500 degrees Fahrenheit (if you get their most expensive ones).

Charcoal grills can get well over 650 degrees and gas grills can get between 600 to 650 degrees.

Of course, charcoal and gas grills also allow for two-zone cooking, where you can leave one side cooler than the other. This lets you grill over direct, very hot heat or indirect, lower heat.

So while you can grill on a Traeger, if you are only going to use it for grilling, you may be better off purchasing a gas or charcoal grill. You may not have as much control over the temperature setting itself, but you have more control over whether you cook with direct or indirect heat.

You can even grill veggies on it, just like you would your traditional grill.

But you don't want to burn them.

Note: You can't actually burn anything in the Traeger. Again, because it uses indirect heat. But you can overcook it. Wood pellet grills produce a varying amount of smoke based on the cooking temperature.

Low temperatures, generally used for smoking, will produce more smoke. High temperatures, like what you'd use for burgers, produce very little smoke.

THE TRICKS AND TIPS TO USING YOUR TRAEGER GRILL

• How do you season a Traeger pellet grill or smoker?

Easy. According to the manual from Traeger, just "Turn the Temperature/Dial to HIGH and run for 45-50 minutes at this setting with the door closed. This must be done before cooking any food on the Grill."
To get specific though, go through these steps which are for the Traeger . You may need to refer to your manual which could have a different procedure:

1. Plug your Traeger in (but keep the power switch off)
2. Put about 1 pound of pellets in the hopper (after checking to make sure it is totally empty)
3. Flip the power switch to on
4. Press any button on the control panel to activate it
5. Press the menu button
6. Turn the dial to auger
7. Select "prime auger"
8. Wait 2 minutes for pellets to move to the firepot
9. Select Back (you don't need that many pellets for seasoning)
10. Turn the dial to set the temp to 350°F
11. Press ignite
12. Close the grill door
13. Run for 20 minutes once it has hit 350°F
14. Turn the dial to set temp to 450°F
15. Run for 30 minutes

16. Initiate the shutdown cycle by pressing and holding the dial for 3 seconds
17. You're done!

The first few times you use your new Traeger, it will prompt you to season it. But you only need to do it once, and that message will eventually stop showing up.

• Smoking in your Traeger

You'll first remove the baffle, drip tray, and grill plates. This will clear the way for any troubleshooting that may need to be done.
Then just put it on the smoke setting.
Then, you want to make sure the auger is spinning. Remember, the auger is what moves the pellets from the hopper to the firepot.
Sometimes during long smoking sessions, the pellets will get stuck to the sides of the hopper. This can be a fire hazard. When the pellets break free, it can lead to "over-firing." Over-firing is the ignition of too many wood pellets at once.
So the hopper will need to be checked periodically, to ensure that there are no pellets stuck to the sides.
This doesn't mean it requires a lot of babysitting like a traditional gas or charcoal grill. It's just something to be aware of.
After you've checked that the auger is spinning, check that air is blowing out of the burner. Do not touch the firepot unless you want to get burned.
Then, put the baffle, grease pan, and grill trays back in the smoker. Fill the pellet box to the top, close the lid, and set the smoker to the desired temperature.

Have patience. Smoking takes time, but it is worth it! Eventually, you'll have delicious, tender, and juicy meat to eat. Gas or charcoal grills can't match the flavor of smoked food!

• How do you preheat a Traeger grill?

Unlike traditional grills, Traeger grills are super easy to preheat.
Really, it's as easy as turning on an oven.
If you've ever used a gas grill, you know that sometimes the pilot light can be a pain to start. Especially if it hasn't been used in a while. If the starter stops working, it can be lit with a long lighter, but it's nerve-wracking to do so. And probably not very safe.
Charcoal is easier to light simply because it doesn't have any starters or hoses that may need bleeding. But you have to be careful with the amount of lighter fluid you use. And it can be a pain to clean up.
By comparison, Traegers are incredibly simple and consistent to light.
When you're ready to cook, just turn the grill on and turn the dial to the "smoke" option. If you have one of the WiFI enabled models, you can even start it from an app on your phone or other smart devices!
If your unit doesn't have a smoke option, set the temperature between 160 and 200 degrees Fahrenheit. Don't put anything on it yet!
Most Trager grills take 10 minutes (or more) to preheat properly. It may take less time depending on the model. Brand new units being fired up will need to be seasoned first (which we get into below).

As the grill is being preheated, you'll hear a roaring noise. That jet engine sound is totally normal. Close the lid to pack in the heat and smoke until the screen shows the temperature you set it to.

Just be aware that unlike an oven, even with the modern advances, the temperature will still vary +/- 20 degrees or so, and that's totally normal.

A Traeger is a wood pellet grill. It uses proprietary wood pellets as fuel. This is different from a wood grill, and especially a charcoal grill.

• How do you use a Traeger for the first time?

To use your Traeger the first time, be sure to refer to Traeger's Owner's Manual.

Unlike traditional grills, your Traeger will need to be plugged into an outlet. It needs power to operate the internal thermostat, fan, igniter rod, and auger. Make sure it is in the off position before you plug it into an outlet.

You can also cover the grease pan with foil for easier cleanup before you put it back in the smoker.

Since this is the first time you're using your Traeger, you'll need to season it first before putting any food in. That takes about 50 minutes, but you only need to do it once. Details on that procedure are further down in my article.

Traeger pellet grills and smokers need to preheat for at least 10 minutes with the door closed before adding any food to it.

But once you've seasoned it, it's just a matter of setting the temp and settings to what you're wanting.

• What should I do if my Traeger runs out of pellets while using it?

Of course, if you have some on hand, it's easy to simply lift the lid and add more to the hopper.

Unfortunately, if you run completely out of pellets during cooking and lose your fire, you have to let the grill cool completely and restart the grill.

Traeger grills use 1-3 pounds of pellets per hour. The hoppers hold between 18 pounds and 22 lbs depending on which model you get.

How fast you go through them, of course, depends on how high your heat is. Pellets are sold in 20-pound bags. Each bag provides between 6 and 20 hours of cook time. The lower the heat, the longer the cooking time you'll need, and the more pellets you'll use.

Some of the best foods are smoked over long periods of time. St. Louis ribs may cook for up to 8 hours. A beef brisket will cook for 12-15 hours.

So for a brisket (yes, please), you can expect to use about 10-15 pounds of pellets over the course of cooking.

• So you want to make sure you have enough wood pellets on hand before you start cooking.

Running out of pellets means that the grill has to cool completely and will have to be restarted according to the Traeger's "Initial Firing Instructions." According to Traeger's Owner's Manual, this means removing baffle, drip tray, and grill plates. You'll want those to be cool before you remove them.

Having to wait until the grill and the components cool completely before firing it back up means that your brisket will have to sit there for several hours. This could permit the growth of harmful bacteria.

You could always throw it in the oven to finish it off. But I think you'll find that the end product is not near as tasty as it would have been if it been cooked on the Traeger the whole time.

• One way to prevent running out of pellets while cooking is to purchase a hopper extender.

Hopper extensions help add 10 pounds of pellets to your hoppers, increasing cooking time by about 25%. Hopper extensions are well priced and bolt right on to the existing hopper. Traeger does not make an extender, but you will find plenty of companies that do.

Just make sure it's designed to fit your model.

How long does a bag of Traeger pellets last?

One of the really neat things about Traeger grills is that they burn real wood, all-natural wood pellets.

The pellets burn in a controlled manner offering convenience and flavor. The pellets are FDA approved and come in a wide variety of flavors. You can even blend the flavors for a unique flavor.

The smoker burns 1-3 pounds of pellets per hour, depending on the temperature you are cooking at. This means each 20-pound bag provides 6 to 20 hours of cooking time.

If you mostly grill, a 20-pound bag could last quite a while. However, if you love to smoke your food, a bag could potentially last for only one or two cooking sessions.

On the low end, Traeger wood pellets are about $18 bucks for a bag. So having multiple bags on hand is a little bit of an investment.

Consider having a variety of flavors on hand, too. But multiple bags on hand means always have enough fuel readily available and lots of flavors to try out.

You don't have to use Traeger wood pellets, although Traeger, of course, recommends that (and if they can prove it, it will void your warranty). But Traeger pellets are actually pretty well priced compared to other brands.

Do make sure to not leave unused pellets in your Traeger for an extended period of time.

Once your Traeger is off and cooled down, simply open the hopper cleanout hatch and let all the unused pellets fall back into the bag. Then just store that bag in a cool, dry place.

Leaving unused pellets in your grill for a long time invites moisture into your pellets which is a bad thing for grilling and smoking.

Do you have to season a pellet smoker?
Yes.

According to the Traeger's Owner's Manual, the smoker must be seasoned before you place any food on the grill.

The grill will need to run on high for 45 minutes with the door closed to be seasoned properly.

Grills need to be seasoned for two reasons.

The first is to burn off any oils and coatings that were introduced during the manufacturing process. You certainly don't want to eat any of that nasty stuff.

The second is to cure the paint. Many paints used in grills generally require high heat to burn off volatiles and form an impermeable barrier.

Seasoning also makes food taste better and will extend the life of your grill. Seasoning isn't just for pellet smokers. Any grill should be seasoned before use.

TRAEGER WOOD PELLET GRILL VS CHARCOAL AND WOOD GRILLS

BENEFITS OF A PELLET GRILL

We already know that pellet grills can be used to smoke, grill, bake and even braise food, and with all those capabilities it's no surprise that they act more like an outdoor oven than a traditional grill. However, the team at Traeger (one of the leading providers of pellet grills) says that most first time users are shocked at the versatility of a pellet grill. Ginevra Iverson, test kitchen director at Food Network, says that with all those capabilities, the options for what to cook on a pellet grill are nearly endless because unlike other grills or smokers, a pellet grill allows you to cook something low and slow — or hotter and faster. You can also set a specific temperature which makes for consistent, efficient cooking every time. Ginevra mentions that with no direct heat cooking and no open flame, you don't even have to worry about flare-ups!

Traeger Pellet Grill vs Gas Grill

The biggest difference between a pellet grill and a gas grill: the flavor! Pellet grills are powered by hardwood pellets and thus impart a naturally sweet, spicy, smoky flavor to everything you cook; a flavor that is unmatched by cooking on gas or charcoal grills. The team at Traeger says: "The smoke acts as a wholly separate seasoning, adding a deeper and more robust flavor to whatever you decide to cook."

Ginevra agrees, and says that the flavor of cooking with wood pellets doesn't even compare to the flavor of cooking on a gas grill. Sure, you can argue that cooking over an open flame like you would on a gas grill gives off flavor, but what if you could get that meaty, smoky flavor without the inevitable ashy, burnt and blackened taste? That's where your pellet grill comes in. Heat is generated through combustion, by igniting wood pellets and circulating heat through a fan system. Much like a convection oven, this allows us to set and maintain a specific temperature without worrying about the unpredictability of open fire flare-ups.

Traeger Pellet Grill vs Charcoal Grill

Although charcoal grills are certainly known for smoky flavor, there's one major difference that sets pellet grills apart from their charcoal counterpart: temperature regulation. Whatever temperature you decide to set your pellet grill to, you can be certain that it will maintain it. One of the biggest downfalls of a charcoal grill is that although it can achieve high temperatures, it's difficult to maintain high temperatures. We've all been there; you've heated your coals to the perfect temperature and before you know it, they're cooling off again! Pellet grills allow you to set a specific cooking temperature (some even support the use of an internal thermometer that pairs with your Bluetooth), so you can check on the doneness of your meat from the comfort of your couch. This system makes for a much more predictable, manageable and convenient grilling experience.

THE WEIRD FOODS YOU CAN COOK WITH YOUR TRAEGER

No amount of frying or conventional cooking can provide you the juicy taste and the satiating sensation of a grilled meal. But do you think your old and worn out grill can compete with the new Traeger Grill? Think again. This remarkable product provides you the smokiest and juiciest meals.

1. The good smoked salmon

There is nothing that can match the temptation of a tender salmon grilled till had an excellent smoky flavor. The recipe for the salmon is simple. Just place your Trager grill on smoke for 4 to 5 minutes and keep the lid open. Then close the lid, set the temperature to 375 degrees and let it preheat for at least 15 minutes.

Take a whole salmon (or fillets if you like) and dip them in a mixture of olive oil, dill, lemon juice, parsley, and garlic. Now place it directly on the grill and let it cook. Once the meat starts to get flaky, take it off the grill and serve with some tantalizing dips or cauliflower pickle salad.

2. Pork tenderloin smoked and served with a veggie casserole

Prepare a marinade with honey, black pepper, thyme, brown sugar and apple juice. Add a few spices of your choice to personalize the recipe. Add the tenderloins to the marinade and let it sit for at least 2 hours. Keep the tenderloin in the refrigerator and allow it absorb all the marinade slowly.

When your friends and family arrive, smoke the grill with the lid open for 5 minutes. Now close the lid and then preheat to 225 degrees for at least 10 minutes. Now place the tenderloins on the grill and let them cook slowly for the next 2 to 3 hours. When fully done, take big slices of the tenderloin and serve with a vegetable casserole. For kids, you can cut smaller pieces. Then butter a small bun, apply some mayonnaise, add the tenderloin piece with fresh veggies and pickles and serve as a burger. If the adults are craving the carbs, pass them one as well.

3. Perfectly smoked marinade brisket

It is very easy to make the brisket wrong. This is why most people go to restaurants to eat this fantastic dish. Don't worry. You can cook it at home as well. Forget about the last time you used a propane grill and made a flaky, overcooked brisket. This is the recipe and the right equipment you will need.

Start by preparing the perfect marinade for the brisket. Take a few garlic cloves and add one teaspoon olive oil to them. Make sure you don't peel the cloves. Just expose their tops by cutting slightly at one end. Now, start your grill and let it smoke for 5 minutes with an open lid. Place the garlic mix on the grill and cook until the cloves are soft. It will take about 30 to 45 minutes for the cloves to soften. Remove from the grill and let cool.

Squeeze the garlic out of the bubs and add 1 cup spicy brown mustard, 2 cups red wine, ½ cup olive oil, ½ cup agave nectar and the brisket rub of your choice. Mix all ingredients properly till you get a smooth consistency. Place the marinade in a large plastic bad, add your brisket and then toss it a little. Let it sit for at least 2 hours, so all flavors are absorbed. You should turn the brisket on the other side after 1 hour.

That's it. Your brisket is now prepared for a smoke session. Preheat the grill and add the brisket after 10 to 15 minutes directly on the grill. Once done, keep cooking for the next 30 minutes. You will be refreshed with the juicy, tender and delicious results. Serve them with the sides of your choice.

THE EASIEST WAY TO FIRE UP YOUR GRILL AND SMOKER

WAYS TO LIGHT YOUR CHARCOAL GRILL THE RIGHT WAY

This first method is one of the simplest ways you can get a large number of briquettes red hot and ready to cook on in just a few minutes.

The Charcoal Method

Using a charcoal chimney starter is the preferred method by most because it works well, is clean and cheap, and is relatively quick compared to lighting the coal from inside your grill.

It's not best for kamado style grills though because of the narrow sides of the grill.

A charcoal "chimney" is nothing but a metal tube that holds your charcoal or briquettes in place while you ignite them from the bottom. The heat rises through the chimney, which sucks more air in from the bottom. So as the coals light, they are effectively 'self-fanning,' as if being blown on all the time, and become lit and hot in a very short time.

You can make your own charcoal chimney starter using a piece of aluminum 6-inch diameter stove pipe.

For most of us who don't have the tools or desire, you can buy a well-constructed chimney in any store that sells grills. They're inexpensive and well worth whatever you pay for one.

Step 1 – Place two sheets of wadded up newspaper in the bottom of the chimney.

Step 2 – Pour in the charcoal or briquettes in the top. Fill the chimney to the top for maximum heat in your grill, or only half way if using the minion method for low and slow cooking.

Step 3 – Place the chimney in the bottom of the grill and light the newspaper.

Step – 4 Once the top layer of coals in the chimney have started to ash over, this is when the coals are ready. So now carefully dump the chimney into the grill and spread them evenly.

Pros:
• Inexpensive
• No chemicals or electricity
• Works every time

Cons:
• The side handle makes it hard to use in deep or narrow grills like the Kamado or Big Green Egg.
The chimney method is the least expensive and adds no chemicals to your fire like some of the other methods.

The Looftlighter Method

The Looftlighter is a combination heater and blower that directs super-heated air toward the charcoal, igniting it in seconds.
Not only will it light a charcoal grill in less than a couple of minutes, but the built-in stand is also a bottle opener. Let's face it, fire starting and bottle opening with one device is pure genius!
If you're unfamiliar with a Looftlighter, you can see it in action in this video by the inventor himself.

Step 1 – Plug in the Looftlighter
Step 2 – Touch the tip of the lighter to the base of the charcoal pile and push the button
Step 3 – Once you see glowing coals or sparks, hold it back about an inch, still pointing at the same spot.

Step 4 – After 60 seconds, the coals should have enough heat to keep burning. Turn it off and open a cold beer with the built-in opener.

Pros:
• The fastest way to light your charcoal or briquettes
• Has a built-in bottle opener
• No chemicals

Cons:
• The most expensive method
• Requires electricity

The Looflighter costs around $80 (as of 11th Nov 2017) or about 13 bottles of lighter fluid.

The two best benefits from this are it is the fastest lighting method and uses no chemicals. The bottle opener is a nice touch too, so long as you don't sear your hand getting the bottle open.

If money is no object, then the Looftlighter is the way to go. It's my preferred method and perfect for any grill, especially Kamado style/ Big Green Egg grills.

Charcoal Starter

This method is also a good way to start your grill without chemicals.

The electric starter is just like an electric stove burner element but bent in a "U" shape with a handle.

It's not as fast or sexy as the Looftlighter, but it will get your fire going. You can see a quick video of the set up here.

Step 1 – Place the burner element in the base of the grill with the handle sticking out.

Step 2 – Pile the charcoal on top

Step 3 – Plug it in.

Step 4 – Once the coals start to glow, unplug the burner and remove it.

This method lights a smaller area of charcoal than the chimney method so it may take longer to get a big fire going if you're grilling over a large area. But if you only need a small fire or just smoking low and slow, this works well.

Pros:
• No chemicals
• Never fails
• Fast

Cons:
• Requires electricity

Electric fire starters work with any type of grill.

Fire Lighter or Fire Starter Method

Fire lighters or starters use paraffin wax, compressed cardboard or wax coated wood shavings to ignite the charcoal. They also work well to start your chimney and don't leave ash as a newspaper will. Also, paraffin wax is non-toxic and doesn't leave any odor or residue.

You will find a variety of brands, in cubes, strips or loosely packed in a box or bag.

You can also make firestarters yourself. Here is a video demonstrating the technique using paper egg cartons and shortening instead of wax. They have a phenomenal 8-minute burn time.

Step 1 – Place the fire starter under the chimney or directly on the pile of charcoal
Step 2 – Light it.
That's all there is to using these to light the coals.

Pros:
• They work well and burn 8 minutes or more if you have wet or stubborn briquettes
• Inexpensive
• Weatherproof

Cons:
• If the flammable agent is chemical, it can affect the taste of your food, so make sure they are labelled 'natural.'
These starters will work in any grill or campfire. Avoid fire starters that use other chemicals besides paraffin wax or vegetable oil. These can taint your cooking with chemical taste if not completely burned.

Paper, Kindling, Charcoal Method

With this method, you build a fire to light your charcoal.

It's more labor intensive and not always reliable. But, if you can do it with one match you might get a merit badge from the Boy Scouts for fire building.

Step 1 – Make a base for your fire by putting down a layer of charcoal or briquettes.

Step 2 – Wad up 2 to 4 sheets of newspaper and place them in the center.

Step 3 – Add thin, dry sticks in a criss-cross pattern over the paper. Press down to make a level surface.

Step 4 – Add some charcoal on top and light the paper.

Step 5 – Once some of the charcoal lights and starts to ash over, add more to build up your fire.

Pros:
• No Chemicals

Cons:
• You need fire building skills, dry kindling wood and patience
• You're making a fire to start a fire
• Slow

This method takes the longest. But you'll get the satisfaction knowing you can build a fire and that you didn't use any lighter fluid or starters.
• Hard to do in wet conditions
• Lighter Fluid Method

We've all used lighter fluid in a pinch. You're in a hurry, or it's raining, and the charcoal is soggy. Lighter fluid is a sure thing.

The trade-off is that it's dangerous and often leaves a petroleum/chemical aftertaste in your food. I recommend you avoid this method for these reasons.

Step 1 – Create a pyramid of briquettes in the bottom of your grill.

Step 2 – Squirt a liberal amount of lighter fluid onto the pile of briquettes, and leave to soak in for a good 30s to a minute. Close the bottle and take it at least 10 feet away from the grill before lighting.

Step 3 – Light the fire using a long matchless lighter or rolled up piece of newspaper. Keep your hands out of the grill in case there is a vapor flash fire.

Never Substitute Gasoline (Petrol) for Charcoal Lighter Fluid.

Yes, the fireball may be spectacular, but the risks outweigh the rewards. Charcoal lighter fluid burns slower and does not have the flammable fumes of gasoline.

Pros:
• It will get any fire going
• It's fast

Cons:
• Dangerous
• Can leave a chemical residue on your food
• Hazardous to store when not using

You can start a fire in any grill with lighter fluid, in almost any conditions. The danger comes when you don't use enough, and it does not light the briquettes. Adding more can make your food taste like petroleum, and it can also cause an explosion. Avoid using lighter fluid for your grill.

TRAEGER GRILL RECIPES

TRAEGER BEEF RECIPES

BEEF TIPS

- Marinate beef for the times directed by the recipe. Do not over-marinate, or the meat can develop a mushy texture.
- For better color and caramelization, knock most of the solid marinade ingredients off meat (garlic, onions, etc.) and dry it thoroughly with paper towels before grilling.
- Season beef just before cooking with your favorite Traeger Rub or Shake or salt and pepper. Otherwise, the salt will begin to draw moisture out of the meat.
- Always let beef rest before carving or serving to allow the natural meat juices redistribute themselves; the time will depend on the cut of meat. Let thinner steaks and hamburgers rest 2

to 3 minutes, thicker cuts 4 to 5 minutes, and brisket, prime rib, or beef shoulder clod, 20 minutes or longer.

- Keep meat refrigerated until you cook it. (The "danger zone" is between 40 and 140 degrees F.) Premium steakhouses never leave their meats out at room temperature.
- Invest in a reliable instant-read or remote meat thermometer and memorize cooking temperatures for rare (125 degrees F), medium-rare (135 to 140 degrees F), and well-done (150 degrees F and above).
- Top steaks with a pat of room-temperature butter before letting them rest for extra flavor and richness.
- Remember that meat will continue to rise several degrees in temperature as it rests.

BARBECUED FLAT IRON STEAKS

A butcher confided to us that flat iron steaks (also known as beef shoul- der top blade steaks) are his favorite cut of beef. Taken from the top of the chuck, they are meaty-tasting, well-marbled, and are best when served medium-rare. Use them the next time you make fajitas.

SERVES: 4
RECOMMENDED PELLETS: Hickory, Mesquite

INGREDIENTS
4 flat iron steaks, each 1/2- to 3/4-inch thick, 7 to 8 ounces each

Traeger beef rub, or your favorite barbecue rub
2 tablespoons minced parsley

DIRECTIONS

1. Season the steaks well on both sides with Traeger Beef Rub. Rub the seasoning in with your fingers.

2. When ready to cook, start the Traeger grill on Smoke with the lid open until the fire is established (4 to 5 minutes). Set the temperature to 450 degrees F (High) and preheat, lid closed, for 10 to 15 minutes.

3. Arrange the steaks on the grill grate and grill, turning once, for 8 to 10 minutes for medium-rare, or 11 to 13 minutes for medium, turning once halfway through grilling.

4. Transfer to a platter or plates and sprinkle with parsley. Let the steaks rest 2 minutes before serving to give the juices a chance to redistribute themselves.

BEEF TENDERLOIN

A two-step cooking process—searing and then roasting on the Traeger—is one of the best ways to handle this pricy, special occasion meat. You can simplify this recipe by skipping the mustard coating, but it does help keep this lean cut moist. An instant-read meat thermometer will help you achieve the perfect degree of doneness.

SERVES: 4-6
RECOMMENDED PELLETS: Oak, Pecan, Hickory

INGREDIENT
2 tablespoons extra- virgin olive oil (divided use)
1 2- to 3-pound filet of beef, trimmed, preferably center cut (see note below)
Traeger beef rub or prime rib rub, or coarse salt and freshly ground black pepper
1/3 cup dijon-style mustard
1 teaspoon dried thyme leaves or 1 tablespoon fresh thyme leaves
1 teaspoon worcestershire sauce

DIRECTIONS

1. Heat a large skillet, preferably cast iron, on the stovetop over medium-high heat. Add one tablespoon of the olive oil to the pan. Season the meat with the Traeger Beef Rub. When the oil is shimmering, put the meat into the pan, searing it well on all sides. (Don't forget the ends: Carefully hold the meat upright with tongs.) Transfer the meat to a rimmed baking sheet. In a small bowl, combine the mustard, thyme, Worcestershire sauce, and the remaining tablespoon of olive oil and mix well. Brush or slather the mustard mixture over the outside of the filet.

2. When ready to cook, start the Traeger grill on Smoke with the lid open until the fire is established (4 to 5 minutes). Set the temperature to 400 degrees F and preheat, lid closed, for 10 to 15 minutes.

3. Put the filet directly on the grill grate and roast for 25 to 30 minutes, or until an instant- read meat thermometer registers an internal temperature of 135 degrees F (for medium- rare). Cook less time if you prefer your meat rarer than that, or more time if you like it well-done. Transfer to a cutting board and let the meat rest, tented with aluminum foil, for 5 minutes before slicing and serving.

Note: If your filet has a narrow "tail" on one end, fold it under the tenderloin and secure it with butcher's string so the tenderloin cooks evenly along its length.

TRAEGER SMOKED T-BONES

A T-bone (and its larger cousin, the Porterhouse) consists of a strip steak and a tenderloin separated by a T-shaped bone. Topping the meat with butter is a trick employed by fancy steakhouses.

SERVES: 4
RECOMMENDED PELLETS:
Hickory, Oak, Mesquite

INGREDIENT
4 T-bone steaks (14- to 16-ounces each), at least 1-inch thick
Your favorite Traeger Rub, or coarse salt and freshly ground black pepper
4 tablespoons butter, at room temperature

DIRECTIONS
1. Season the steaks on both sides with the Traeger Rub.

2. When ready to cook, start the Traeger grill on Smoke with the lid open until the fire is established (4 to 5 minutes).

3. Arrange the steaks on the grill grate and smoke for 30 minutes.

4. Set the temperature to 450 degrees F (High), and preheat, lid closed, for 10 to 15 minutes. Cook the steaks to your desired degree of doneness, turning once, about 15 to 20 minutes for medium-rare (135 degrees F), longer if you prefer your steaks more done. Top each with a pat of butter. Let the steaks rest for 3 minutes before carving and serving.

BETTER BURGERS

In recent years, we've been challenged to cook beef burgers to a safe internal temperature of 160 degrees F without drying them out. That's a difficult order on a conventional grill, but easy on a Traeger. The gentle indirect heat cooks the meat through and leaves it juicy as all get out.

SERVES: 4
RECOMMENDED PELLETS: Hickory, Oak, Mesquite

INGREDIENT
2 pounds ground chuck, 80/20 or 85/15 (lean to fat ratio)
2 teaspoons traeger beef rub, or substitute your favorite barbecue rub
1 cup mayonnaise (preferably hellmann's)
1/4 cup traeger regular barbecue sauce, or your favorite barbecue sauce

3 tablespoons butter, melted
4 kaiser rolls, split
Lettuce leaves
Sweet onion slices
Tomato slices
Dill pickle chips

DIRECTIONS

1. Make sure the meat is well-chilled before handling. Combine the ground beef and Traeger Beef Rub in a medium bowl. Wet your hands with cold water, and mix gently. Divide the meat into four equal portions. Rewet your hands with cold water, and form each portion into a patty about 4 inches in diameter and 3/4-inch thick. (Try not to overwork the meat.) Using your thumbs, make a shallow wide depression on the top of each burger. (This prevents the burger from developing a bulge in the middle.)

2. Combine the mayonnaise and the barbecue sauce in a shallow bowl and refrigerate until serving time.

3. Brush the cut sides of the kaiser rolls with the melted butter.

4. When ready to cook, start the Traeger grill on Smoke with the lid open until the fire is established (4 to 5 minutes). Set the
temperature to 425 degrees F and preheat, lid closed, for 10 to 15 minutes.

5. Arrange the burgers directly on the grill grate, depression-side down. Cook for 10 minutes, then flip. Cook for 10 to 15 minutes more, or until an instant-read meat thermometer (put the probe through the side of the burger) registers 160 degrees F.

6. Meanwhile, lightly toast the buns, cut sides down. Watch carefully as buttered bread can easily burn.

7. Spread the cut sides of the buns with the mayonnaise sauce. Put a burger on each bun bottom, and top with lettuce, onion, tomato, and pickle. Finish with the top of the bun. Serve immediately.

PRIME RIB WITH HORSERADISH CREAM

Prime rib is, of course, one of the most luxurious cuts of beef you can buy. And it's amazing when roasted on a Traeger. A remote meat thermometer is a real help when cooking a large, bone-in roast like prime rib. It will eliminate the need to lift the grill lid frequently to check on your investment. Remember that the roast will continue to cook as it rests, so take it off the grill when it is 5 to 10 degrees cooler than your desired serving temperature.

SERVES: 6-8
RECOMMENDED PELLETS:
Hickory, Oak, Pecan

INGREDIENT
One 3-to-4-pound prime rib
Traeger Prime Rib or Beef Rub, or equal parts of kosher salt and coarsely ground black pepper

Granulated garlic (optional)
Horseradish Cream (recipe follows)
Large roasting pan with a meat rack
Butcher's string

DIRECTIONS

1. Allow the roast to come to room temperature before grilling. Tie it at intervals with butcher's string. (This keeps it from separating along the inner fat line as it cooks.) Season the roast well with the Traeger Prime Rib or Beef Rub, or the salt/
pepper mixture. Sprinkle with the granulated garlic, if desired. Use your fingers to pat the seasonings into the meat. Place the meat rack in the roasting pan; put the roast, bone-side down and uncovered, on the rack.

2. When ready to cook, start the Traeger grill on Smoke with the lid open until the fire is established (4 to 5 minutes). Set the temperature to 450 degrees F (High) and preheat, lid closed, for 10 to 15 minutes.

3. Roast for 30 minutes. Reduce the temperature to 300 degrees F, and continue to cook until the internal temperature in the thickest part of the meat reads 130 degrees F (for medium-rare) as read on an instant-read meat thermometer. (Figure on roughly 18 to 20 minutes per pound total cooking time.)

4. Allow the prime rib to rest for 20 minutes. Remove the butcher's string. Transfer the meat to a large cutting board. With a sharp knife, carve off the rack of bones and put them aside for gnawing. Slice the meat and serve immediately with the Horseradish Cream (see below).

5. Horseradish Cream: Combine 1-1/2 Cups sour cream, 1/4 cup prepared horseradish (or more to taste), 1 tablespoon Dijon mustard, 1 teaspoon Worcestershire sauce, and salt and pepper to taste. Refrigerate, covered, until ready to serve.

BEGINNER'S BRISKET

Brisket is a cut from between a steer's forelegs. It is a muscle used frequently by the animal, which explains its beefy flavor and its need to be cooked low and slow for hours. Look for a brisket with a cap of fat at least 1/4-inch thick. Allow more time than you think you'll need as every brisket is different. And always bring it to an internal temperature of 190 to 195 degrees F for maximum tenderness. Baked beans are a great accompaniment.

SERVES: 10-12
RECOMMENDED PELLETS:
Hickory, Oak

INGREDIENT
1 6-pound brisket flat, trimmed
Traeger Beef Rub, or your favorite barbecue rub
Cups beef broth, beer, or cola
1/4 cup apple cider vinegar
2 tablespoons Worcestershire sauce
Traeger Texas Spicy Barbecue Sauce, or your favorite barbecue sauce

DIRECTIONS
1. Season the brisket on both sides with the Traeger Beef Rub. Make the mop sauce: In a clean spray bottle, combine the beef broth, beer, or cola with the vinegar and Worcestershire sauce.

2. When ready to cook, start the Traeger grill on Smoke with the lid open until the fire is established (4 to 5 minutes). Arrange the brisket fat-side up on the grill grate and smoke for 3 to 4 hours, spraying with the mop sauce every hour. Set the temperature to 225 degrees F and continue to cook the brisket, spraying occasionally with mop sauce, until an instant-read thermometer inserted in the thickest part of the meat reads 190 to 195 degrees F. (This will likely take 4 to 6 hours more, or even longer. Be patient and don't rush the process.)

3. Foil the meat and let it rest for 30 minutes, preferably in an insulated container lined with thick bath towels or newspapers so the meat stays hot. Slice with a sharp knife across the grain into pencil-width slices. Serve the barbecue sauce separately on the side.

LONE STAR BARBECUED BRISKET

Brisket is one tough cut of meat. Above all, it requires patience on the part of the barbecuer. It may take it some time to get from 150 degrees F to 190 degrees F, a period known as a "plateau". Do not be tempted to turn the heat up at this point. If your brisket is tender before your guests arrive, wrap it tightly in foil, then thick towels and let it rest in an insulated cooler. It will stay hot for more than an hour. You can also rewarm foil-wrapped brisket on your Traeger or in your oven (275 to 300 degrees F).

SERVES: 8-10
RECOMMENDED PELLETS:
Oak, Mesquite

INGREDIENT
1 Cup cold brewed coffee
1 Cup Texas beer
2 tablespoons brown sugar
1 tablespoon chile powder
1 teaspoon garlic salt
1/4 cup Traeger Prime Rib Rub
1 tablespoon ground coffee
4- to 5-pound center- cut brisket flat, trimmed
Traeger Texas Spicy Barbecue Sauce
9x13-inch aluminum foil disposable pan
Aluminum foil
A clean spray bottle

DIRECTIONS
1. Make the mop sauce: Combine the coffee, beer, brown sugar, chile powder and garlic salt in a bowl and whisk to dissolve any salt or sugar crystals. Transfer to a clean spray bottle and set aside.

2. In a small bowl, mix the Traeger Prime Rib Rub and the ground coffee. Rub this mixture on the brisket, covering all surfaces.

3. When ready to cook, start the Traeger grill on Smoke with the lid open until the fire is established (4 to 5 minutes).

4. Put the brisket directly on the grill grate and smoke for 2 hours. Spray the brisket with the mop sauce and transfer to a disposable aluminum foil pan. Increase the temperature to 275 degrees F and continue to cook for 4 to 5 hours, spraying every hour with the mop sauce. If at any point the brisket appears to be drying out, cover it tightly with aluminum foil. (Discontinue mopping if you do this.) When done, the internal temperature of the brisket will be 185 to 190 degrees F (anything less, and your brisket will be tough). Let rest for 20 to 30 minutes before carving against the grain (see Note below) into pencil-thick slices. Serve, if desired, with barbecue sauce on the side. Good accompaniments include baked beans and biscuits or cornbread.

SMOKED CORNED BEEF BRISKET

Once you've tasted corned beef cooked in its own juices on your Traeger, you'll never go back to boiled corned beef again. And leftovers, if you have any, make terrific Reuben sandwiches.

SERVES: 6-8
RECOMMENDED PELLETS:
Hickory, Oak, Apple, Pecan

INGREDIENT
1 Corned beef brisket flat, 3 to 4 pounds, with a fat cap at least 1/4 inch thick
1 bottle Traeger Apricot Barbecue Sauce, or your favourite fruit-based barbecue sauce

1/4 cup Dijon-style mustard

DIRECTIONS

1. Remove the corned beef brisket from its packaging and discard the spice packet, if any.

2. When ready to cook, start the Traeger grill on Smoke with the lid open until the fire is established (4 to 5 minutes). Set the temperature to 275 degrees F and preheat, lid closed, for 10 to 15 minutes.

3. Put the corned beef brisket directly on the grill grate, fat side up, and cook for 2 hours. Meanwhile, combine the barbecue sauce and the mustard in a medium bowl, whisking to mix.

4. Pour half of the barbecue sauce-mustard mixture in the bottom of a disposable aluminum foil pan. With tongs, transfer
the brisket to the pan, fat-side up. Pour the remainder of the barbecue sauce-mustard mixture over the top of the brisket, using a spatula to spread the sauce evenly. Cover the pan tightly with aluminum foil. Return the brisket to the grill and continue to cook for 2 to 3 hours, or until the brisket is tender. The internal temperature should be 185 degrees F on an instant-read meat thermometer. Allow the meat to rest for 15 to 20 minutes.

5. Slice across the grain into 1/4-INCh slices with a sharp knife and serve immediately. If desired, spoon some of the sauce over each serving.

BEEF JERKY

Very lean meat, cut across the grain, makes the best jerky. Be sure to trim out any fat or connective tissue you see when you're preparing the meat. Because some moisture will be left in the jerky at the end of the smoking time, refrigerate the meat for longer-term storage.

SERVES: 12
RECOMMENDED PELLETS:
Hickory, Oak, Pecan

INGREDIENTS
1/2 Cup soy sauce
1/2 Cup beer, cola, or water
1/4 cup Worcestershire sauce
2 teaspoons garlic powder
1 teaspoon onion powder
1 teaspoon freshly ground black pepper
2 pounds trimmed beef top or bottom round, sirloin tip, or flank steak

DIRECTIONS
1. In a mixing bowl, combine the soy sauce, water, Worcestershire sauce, garlic powder, onion powder, and pepper and whisk to mix.

2. With a sharp knife, slice the beef into 1/4- inch thick slices against the grain. (This is easier if the meat is partially frozen.) Trim any fat or connective tissue. Put the beef slices in a large resealable plastic bag. Pour the soy sauce mixture over the beef, and massage the bag so that all the slices get coated with the marinade. Seal the bag and refrigerate for several hours, or overnight.

3. When ready to cook, start the Traeger grill on Smoke with the lid open until the fire is established (4 to 5 minutes).

4. Remove the beef from the marinade and discard the marinade. Dry the beef slices between paper towels. Arrange the meat in a single layer directly on the grill grate.

5. Smoke for 4 to 5 hours, or until the jerky is dry but still chewy and somewhat pliant when you bend a piece. Transfer to a resealable plastic bag while the jerky's still warm. Let the jerky rest for an hour at room temperature. Squeeze any air from the bag, and refrigerate the jerky. It will keep for several weeks.

FILETS MIGNONS

Cut from the small end of a whole beef tenderloin, filets mignons are perfect for a dinner for two. Try to buy steaks that are at least an inch thick if you prefer your filets rare or medium-rare. Though it's optional, you can wrap a strip of bacon around the outside of each filet before cooking for a fancier presentation. Mushrooms sautéed with butter, garlic, and a splash of Worcestershire sauce make a nice side dish.

SERVES: 2
RECOMMENDED PELLETS:
Alder, Oak, Pecan

INGREDIENTS

2 filets mignons, each about 1-1/4 inch thick
Traeger Prime Rib Rub, or coarse salt and freshly ground black pepper

DIRECTIONS
1. Season the steaks with the Traeger Prime Rib Rub, patting it on with your fingertips.

2. When ready to cook, start the Traeger grill on Smoke with the lid open until the fire is established (4 to 5 minutes). Set the temperature to 450 degrees F (High) and preheat, lid closed, for 10 to 15 minutes.

3. Arrange the steaks on the grill grate. Cook for 7 minutes. Turn with tongs, and cook for 5 to 7 minutes more, or until the internal temperature reaches 135 degrees F on an instant-read meat thermometer inserted through the side toward the center of the steak. (Adjust the time if you prefer your meat more well-done.) Transfer to a platter or plates and let rest for 2 minutes before serving.

FLANK STEAK

Flank steak comes from a muscle that gets quite a workout, giving it great flavor. But unless it's properly cooked and sliced, it can be a tough chew. The key is to marinate it, cook it to medium-rare, and then slice it thinly on a diagonal across the grain. Leftovers make terrific sandwiches.

SERVES: 4-6
RECOMMENDED PELLETS:
Hickory, Mesquite, Oak

INGREDIENT
1 flank steak, 1-1/2 to 2 pounds
1/2 cup vegetable oil or extra-virgin olive oil
1/4 cup red wine vinegar
1 tablespoon dijon-style mustard
1/2 onion, sliced
1 clove garlic, minced
Traeger Beef Rub or Prime Rib Rub, or salt and freshly ground black pepper

DIRECTIONS
1. In a small bowl, whisk together the oil, vinegar, and mustard.

2. Lay the flank steak in a baking dish large enough to hold it. Season the flank steak on both sides with the Traeger Beef Rub, patting the seasoning down with your fingertips.
Pour the oil mixture over it, turning to coat, then top with the onions and garlic. Marinate, covered with plastic wrap and refrigerated, for 4 to 8 hours, turning once.

3. When ready to cook, start the Traeger grill on Smoke with the lid open until the fire is established (4 to 5 minutes). Set the temperature to 450 degrees F (High) and preheat, lid closed, for 10 to 15 minutes.

4. Lift the flank steak from the marinade (discard the marinade and solids) and pat dry with paper towels. Arrange the steak at a diagonal directly on the grill grate. Grill for 6 minutes, then turn. Continue grilling for 6 to 8 minutes more. (The exact time will depend on the thickness of your steak.) Transfer the steak to a cutting board and let rest for 5 minutes. Reseason with Traeger Beef Rub, if desired. Slice thinly on the diagonal across the grain. Serve immediately.

LONDON BROIL

If you like your meat well-done, this is not the recipe for you. London Broil is best served rare to medium-rare. By the way, London Broil is not a certain cut of meat—rather, it is a cooking method. The meat itself can be several things, including top round, chuck steak, flank steak, or even beef tenderloin.

SERVES: 6-8
RECOMMENDED PELLETS:
Hickory, Oak

INGREDIENTS
2-1/2 to 3-pound beef top round shoulder

Traeger Carne Asada Marinade, or your favorite beef marinade

DIRECTIONS

1. Put the beef and the Traeger Carne Asada Marinade in a large resealable plastic bag. Turn to coat. Refrigerate for several hours, or overnight.

2. When ready to cook, start the Traeger grill on Smoke with the lid open until the fire is established (4 to 5 minutes). Set the temperature to 450 degrees F (High) and preheat, lid closed, for 10 to 15 minutes.

3. Remove the meat from the marinade.
If desired, pour the marinade in a small saucepan and bring to a boil over high heat. Boil for two minutes, then remove from the heat. Strain, and let cool. Now you can use the marinade as a sauce. Keep warm.

4. Pat the meat dry with paper towels. Put the meat on the grill grate and grill 8 to 10 minutes per side, turning once with tongs, or until an instant-read meat thermometer inserted into the thickest part reads 135 degrees F for rare. (Grill a few minutes longer if you prefer your London Broil medium-rare.) Let the meat rest for 3 minutes before slicing thinly on a diagonal against the grain. Serve the warmed marinade as a sauce, if desired.

TRAEGER BEEF ROAST

Just like Mom used to make—if Mom had had a Traeger! Feel free to cook potatoes, carrots, and onions alongside the roast if desired. Chill any leftovers, slice thinly, and use to construct au jus sandwiches.

SERVES: 6-8
RECOMMENDED PELLETS:
Hickory, Oak, Pecan

INGREDIENTS
1 beef chuck, rump, or sirloin tip roast, 3 to 3-1/2 pounds
2 tablespoons vegetable oil or extra-virgin olive oil
Traeger Beef Shake or Rub or Prime Rib Rub, or salt and coarse black pepper
2 Cups beef broth

DIRECTIONS
1. Rub the roast on all sides with the oil and place on a rack in a roasting pan, fat-side up. Season well with the Traeger Beef Shake. Pour the beef broth in the bottom of the pan.

2. When ready to cook, start the Traeger grill on Smoke with the lid open until the fire is established (4 to 5 minutes). Set the temperature to 450 degrees F (High) and preheat, lid closed, for 10 to 15 minutes.

3. Cook the roast for 25 to 30 minutes, or until the outside is seared. Reduce the temperature to 225 degrees F and continue cooking, 2 to 3 hours, or until medium-rare (135 degrees F on an instant-read meat thermometer). Let it reach 155 degrees F if you prefer your meat well-done. Tent the roast with aluminum foil and let the meat rest for 10 minutes before slicing across the grain into thin slices. Serve with the pan drippings, if desired.

BEEF RIBS

Meaty beef long bones—also called beef back ribs, spare ribs, or Texas ribs—can be difficult to find. Butchers usually trim the meat as close to the bone as possible in order to maximize the poundage of boneless prime rib roast and/or rib-eye steaks they can sell. So the next time you splurge on a prime rib roast, ask the butcher to split the difference by leaving more meat on the bones. (Sometimes, they'll do this even if you don't buy the whole prime rib!) These ribs are not to be confused with beef chuck ribs, also called "dinosaur" bones.

SERVES: 4-6
RECOMMENDED PELLETS:
Oak, Hickory
 INGREDIENTS
2 7-bone racks beef long ribs (back ribs), 5 to 6 pounds total
Traeger Prime Rib Rub, or your favorite barbecue rub

Traeger Texas Spicy Barbecue Sauce, or your favorite barbecue sauce

DIRECTIONS

1. If your butcher has not already done so, remove the thin papery membrane from the bone-side of the ribs by working the tip of a butter knife or a screwdriver underneath the membrane over a middle bone. Use paper towels to get a firm grip, then tear the membrane off.

2. Season the ribs with Traeger Prime Rib Rub.

3. When ready to cook, start the Traeger grill on Smoke with the lid open until the fire is established (4 to 5 minutes). Smoke the ribs, meat-side up, for 2 hours. Set the temperature to 225 degrees F.

4. Continue to cook the ribs for 3 to 4 hours more, or until the meat is tender. If desired, wrap the ribs tightly in foil partway through the cooking time. The last 30 minutes, carefully remove the ribs from the foil and brush them liberally with Traeger Texas Spicy Barbecue Sauce, and return to grill. Transfer the ribs to a cutting board and let them rest for a few minutes before carving them into individual ribs.

SANTA MARIA-STYLE TRI-TIP

Until recently, few people outside the Santa Maria Valley in Central Califor- nia were aware of tri-tip, a triangular muscle from the bottom of the sirloin. But its beefy flavor is catching on in other parts of the country. Sometimes, you'll find it sliced into steaks. It is traditionally served medium-rare with fresh salsa, pinquito beans, French bread, and a green salad.

SERVES: 4-6
RECOMMENDED PELLETS: Oak

INGREDIENTS
1 tri-tip roast, 1-1/2 to 2 pounds
Traeger Beef Rub or 1-1/2 teaspoons each salt, freshly ground black pepper, and garlic powder

DIRECTIONS
1. Season the meat well on all sides with the Traeger Beef Rub.

2. When ready to cook, start the Traeger grill on Smoke with the lid open until the fire is established (4 to 5 minutes). Set the temperature to 425 degrees F and preheat, lid closed, for 10 to 15 minutes.

3. Lay the tri-tip directly on the grill grate and cook for 45 to 50 minutes. (Do not overcook or the tri-tip with be tough and dry.) Transfer to a cutting board and tent with aluminum foil. Let the tri-tip rest for 15 minutes before carving across the grain into broad, thin slices.

CHILI-GLAZED MEATLOAF

Meatloaf makes a great Sunday night supper. (Hopefully, you'll have leftovers for Monday sandwiches.) A row of chopped whole carrots in the loaf pan acts like a natural meat rack and keeps the bottom of the meatloaf from getting crusty.

SERVES: 4
RECOMMENDED PELLETS:
Apple, Oak

INGREDIENTS
1-1/2 pounds ground beef
1/2 pound ground pork
1 cup dried bread crumbs
1/4 cup finely minced onion
1 tablespoon traeger cajun rub, or your favorite barbecue rub
1 teaspoon garlic powder
2 eggs
1/2 cup milk
2 teaspoons worcestershire sauce
2 whole carrots, peeled, trimmed, cut into lengths the width of your loaf pan
1/2 cup traeger chili sauce, or your favorite chili sauce

DIRECTIONS
1. In a large mixing bowl, combine the ground beef, ground pork, bread crumbs, onion, Traeger Cajun Rub, and the garlic powder. In another bowl, beat the eggs lightly.

2. Add milk and Worcestershire sauce. Add the liquid ingredients to the meat mixture, and mix with your hands. Lay a few of the carrot pieces down in the loaf pan; the carrots will become a natural rack for the meat. Form the meat into a loaf shape and lay it on top of the carrots.

3. When ready to cook, start the Traeger grill on Smoke with the lid open until the fire is established (4 to 5 minutes). Set the temperature to 350 degrees F and preheat, lid closed, for 10 to 15 minutes.

4. Put the loaf pan on the grill rack. Bake the meatloaf for 50 to 60 minutes, or until the internal temperature reads 160 degrees F when read on an instant-read meat thermometer. Spread the Traeger Chili Sauce on top of the meatloaf the last 10 minutes of cooking. Transfer the meatloaf to a cooling rack and let cool for 10 minutes. Carefully remove it from the loaf pan. (Discard the carrots.) Slice into 1/2-INCh slices for serving.

GAUCHO-STYLE BEEF SHOULDER TENDERS WITH CHIMICHURRI SAUCE

Beef shoulder tenders are an inexpensive alternative to pricy beef tenderloin. Also called "butcher's steak"—which gives you an indication of how good this cut is since butchers used to set it aside for themselves—this long, slender muscle from the shoulder chuck is both lean and beefy-tasting. In the below preparation, the meat is seasoned simply, then grilled over high heat until medium-rare—just as they would do it in South America—and served with chimichurri sauce, sometimes referred to as "Argentinean steak sauce."

SERVES: 3-4
RECOMMENDED PELLETS:
Mesquite, Hickory

INGREDIENTS
2 beef shoulder tenders, 10 to 12 ounces each
Traeger Beef Rub, or coarse salt and freshly ground black pepper
1/4 cup fresh parsley leaves, coarsely chopped
3 cloves garlic, coarsely chopped
2 teaspoons dried oregano
1 teaspoon dried red pepper flakes, or more to taste
1/4 cup red wine vinegar
Salt and freshly ground black pepper to taste
1/2 cup extra-virgin olive oil

DIRECTIONS

1. Season the shoulder tenders with Traeger Beef Rub and set aside.

2. Make the chimichurri: In a blender jar or small food processor, combine the parsley, garlic, oregano, dried red pepper flakes, and red wine vinegar. Pulse until blended. Add salt and pepper to taste. Let the mixture sit for 20 minutes for the flavors to develop. Then slowly blend in the olive oil.

3. When ready to cook, start the Traeger grill on Smoke with the lid open until the fire is established (4 to 5 minutes). Set the temperature to 450 degrees F (High) and preheat, lid closed, for 10 to 15 minutes.

4. Arrange the shoulder tenders on the grill grate. Turn after 10 minutes to put grill marks on the other side. Grill to the desired degree of doneness, 5 to 10 minutes more for medium-rare (135 degrees F on an instant- read meat thermometer).

5. Transfer the meat to a cutting board and let it rest for 3 minutes. Carve it on a diagonal into slices 3/4-inch thick. If desired, pour some of the chimichurri over the meat and serve the rest of the sauce on the side. Or serve the sauce separately.

SOUTHWESTERN POT ROAST

Braised until it's falling-apart-tender, you can serve this over rice or in a tortilla or taco shells.

SERVES: 4-6
RECOMMENDED PELLETS:
Mesquite, Oak, Hickory

INGREDIENTS
3- to 4-pound boneless chuck roast
Traeger fajita rub, or salt and freshly ground black pepper
2 tablespoons oil
1 large onion, peeled and coarsely chopped
2 cloves garlic, minced
1 cup beef broth
10-ounce can diced tomatoes with green chiles
2 teaspoons chile powder, or more to taste
1 teaspoon dried oregano, preferably mexican
1 teaspoon cumin

DIRECTIONS

1. Generously season the roast on all sideswith the Traeger Fajita Rub.

2. Heat a large skillet over medium-high heat. Add the oil. When the oil shimmers, sear the roast on all sides. Transfer the roast to a lidded casserole or baking dish large enough to hold it. Reduce the heat to medium and add the onions, stirring occasionally. Cook for 5 minutes, or until the onions begin to soften. Add the garlic and cook for 2 minutes more.
Add the beef broth, stirring to scrape up the brown bits from the bottom of the pan. Then add the tomatoes, chile powder, oregano, and cumin and bring to a simmer. Add salt and pepper to taste. Tip the onion-tomato mixture over the meat. Put the lid on the casserole.
If using a baking pan, cover it tightly with aluminum foil.

3. When ready to cook, start the Traeger grill on Smoke with the lid open until the fire is established (4 to 5 minutes). Set the
temperature to 250 degrees F and preheat, lid closed, for 10 to 15 minutes.
4. Put the casserole or pan on the grill grate. Roast until the meat is very tender, 3 to 4 hours. (Be careful when lifting the casserole lid or foil as steam will escape.) Slice and serve with the tomato-onion gravy.

"SECRET INGREDIENT" BEEF SHORT RIBS

Traeger Chili Sauce combined with root beer and onions makes a delicious braising sauce for beef short ribs.

SERVE: 4-6
RECOMMENDED PELLETS:
Oak, Hickory, Apple

INGREDIENTS
1 bottle Traeger Chili Barbecue Sauce, or your favorite chili sauce
1 Cup good-quality root beer soda, such as Dr. Brown's or Hane's, plus more as needed
1 tablespoon fresh thyme leaves, chopped
1 large sweet onion, thinly sliced into rings
3 to 4 pounds bone- in short ribs, or 2-1/2 pounds of boneless short ribs
Salt
Freshly ground black pepper
A 9x13-inch aluminum foil disposable baking pan or other baking pan
Aluminum foil

DIRECTIONS
1. In a medium bowl, combine the Traeger Chili Barbecue Sauce, the root beer, and the thyme leaves.

2. Arrange the onions evenly in the bottom of the pan. Season the short ribs on all sides with salt and pepper. Lay in a single layer
on top of the onions. Pour the chili-root beer sauce evenly over the ribs. Cover the pan tightly with aluminum foil.

3. When ready to cook, start the Traeger grill on Smoke with the lid open until the fire is established (4 to 5 minutes). Set the
temperature to 300 degrees F and preheat, lid closed, for 10 to 15 minutes.

4. Put the pan of ribs on the grill grate and cook for 2-1/2 to 3 hours, or until the ribs are tender but not falling off the bone. Add a bit more root beer to the pan if the dish doesn't seem saucy enough. Serve immediately with polenta or mashed potatoes. Short ribs render a fair amount of fat, so if it concerns you, refrigerate the ribs in the sauce overnight. The fat will have solidified on top, and can be removed and discarded before reheating the ribs.

KOREAN BARBECUED SHORT RIBS (KALBI)

If you can't find crosscut beef short ribs, feel free to substitute another cut of beef, such as sirloin or chuck, sliced 1/4-inch thick across the grain. The marinade is also excellent on rib-eyes, skirt steak, and even chicken thighs or breasts.

SERVES: 4
RECOMMENDED PELLETS:
Oak, Pecan, Hickory

INGREDIENTS
1/2 Cup soy sauce
1/2 Cup water
2 tablespoons white vinegar or rice vinegar
2 tablespoons brown sugar
1 tablespoon granulated sugar or honey
2 Cloves garlic, minced
1 ripe pear, peeled, cored, and coarsely chopped
1-inch piece fresh ginger, peeled and sliced into coins
1 scallion (green onion), trimmed and coarsely chopped
2 teaspoons sesame oil
1 teaspoon Traeger Beef Shake, or salt
1-1/2 pounds crosscut beef short ribs (flanken), or see substitutions above

DIRECTIONS

1. Make the marinade: Combine the soy sauce, water, vinegar, brown sugar, granulated sugar, garlic, pear, ginger, scallion, and sesame oil in a blender and pulse several times. Lay the beef in a single layer in a baking dish and season on both sides with Traeger Beef Shake. Pour the marinade over the beef, turning the beef over to coat both sides. Cover and refrigerate for several hours, or overnight.

2. When ready to cook, start the Traeger grill on Smoke with the lid open until the fire is established (4 to 5 minutes). Set the temperature to 450 degrees F (High) and preheat, lid closed, for 10 to 15 minutes.

3. Remove the beef from the marinade; discard marinade. Arrange the beef on the grill grate and grill, 2 to 3 minutes per side, or until the meat is cooked to your liking. (In Korea, they prefer their short ribs well-done.) Transfer to a platter or plates and serve immediately.

SMOKED ITALIAN MEATBALL SUBS

These sandwiches are for hearty appetites—perfect for game day or a busy weeknight supper. You can also form the meat mixture into cocktail-size meatballs (use mini muffin tins to bake them for approximately 20 minutes) and serve on toothpicks with warm marinara as a dipping sauce.

SERVES: 4

INGREDIENT
1-1/2 pounds ground beef
1/2 pound bulk italian sausage or ground pork
3/4 cup seasoned dry bread crumbs
1/2 cup grated parmesan
1/4 cup onion, finely minced
2 cloves garlic, finely minced
1 egg, lightly beaten
1/4 cup milk
2 teaspoons Traeger Beef Rub, or 1 teaspoon each salt and freshly ground black pepper
Your favorite jarred spaghetti or marinara sauce
4 hoagie or sub rolls, split through the side

DIRECTIONS
1. Put all the meatball ingredients (except the spaghetti sauce and rolls) in a large mixing bowl and work the meat mixture with your hands to combine.

2. When ready to cook, start the Traeger grill on Smoke with the lid open until the fire is established (4 to 5 minutes). Set the temperature to 325 degrees F and preheat, lid closed, for 10 to 15 minutes.

3. Bake the meatballs for 30 to 35 minutes, or until they are cooked through. (An instant-read meat thermometer should read 160 degrees F.) Meanwhile, warm the spaghetti sauce in a large frying pan over medium-low heat. Transfer the cooked meatballs to the sauce; keep warm. Put three or 4 meatballs on each roll and top with a few spoonfuls of sauce. Serve immediately.

SMOKED PEPPERED BEEF JERKY
SERVES: 4
Spiced up, irresistible beef jerky. This jerky is doused in a beer, soy sauce and black pepper marinade, and smoked low and slow for an epic protein-packed snack.

INGREDIENTS
1 Bottle dark beer
1 Cup soy sauce
1/4 Cup Worcestershire sauce
3 Tablespoon brown sugar
1 Tablespoon Morton Tender Quick Home Meat Cure
1/2 Teaspoon garlic salt
4 Tablespoon coarse ground black pepper, divided
2 Pound trimmed beef top or bottom round.
2 Tablespoon coarse ground black pepper, divided

DIRECTIONS

Plan ahead, this recipe marinates overnight.

In a mixing bowl, combine the beer, soy sauce, Worcestershire sauce, brown sugar, curing salt, garlic salt and 2 tablespoons of the black pepper.

With a sharp knife, trim any fat or connective tissue off of meat. Slice the beef into 1/4 inch thick slices against the grain (this is easier if the meat is partially frozen).

Put the beef slices into a large resealable plastic bag. Pour the marinade mixture over the beef and massage the bag so that all the slices get coated with the marinade. Seal the bag and refrigerate for several hours to overnight.

When ready to cook, set Traeger temperature to 180°F and preheat, lid closed for 15 minutes. For optimal flavor, use Super Smoke if available.

Grill: 180°

Remove beef slices from the marinade and discard the marinade.

Dry the beef slices between paper towels then sprinkle beef slices generously on both sides with black pepper.

Arrange the meat in a single layer directly on the grill grate. Smoke for 4 to 5 hours or until the jerky is dry but still chewy and somewhat pliant when you bend a piece.

Grill: 180°

Transfer to a resealable plastic bag while the jerky is still warm. Let the jerky rest for an hour at room temperature with the bag open.

Squeeze any air from the bag, seal and refrigerate the jerky. It will keep for several weeks. Enjoy!

TRAEGER PORK RECIPES

THE PORK RECIPE TIPS

- Generally speaking, bone-in meat will have more flavor than boneless cuts.
- Always remove the thin membrane on the back of a rack of ribs to increase smoke and spice absorption. (Use a the tip of a screwdriver or butter knife to get
- Under the membrane, then grip it and pull it off with a paper towel.)
- Grill or smoke meat with the fat cap facing up.
- For extra flavor, drape leaner cuts of pork (such as tenderloin or pork loin roast) with slices of bacon while cooking.
- Tuck a pan of apple juice into a corner of the Traeger to keep meat moist during long cooks (especially good with ribs). Alternatively, transfer the juice to a clean spray bottle and periodically mist the meat. Remember that

lifting the lid will add to your total cooking time.

- Like poultry, pork sometimes benefits from brining before cooking.
- Apply barbecue sauce the last few minutes of cooking to "set" the sauce and avoid scorching it. (Most sauces are high in sugars, which have a tendency to burn on the grill.)
- A pinkish ring just below the surface of the meat (and sometimes on the bone as well) is called a "smoke ring," and is the sign of a smoking job well done!
- If grilling chops rimmed with a layer of fat, make small vertical cuts in the fat to discourage it from curling as the chops cook.

3-2-1 BABY BACK RIBS

The 3-2-1 method of barbecuing ribs—3 hours of smoke, 2 hours wrapped tightly in foil, and 1 hour sauced—has become very popular among competition barbecuers and home cooks alike, especially those who prefer their ribs "fall-off-the-bone" tender. Adjust the cooking time if you like your ribs with more chew. Feel free to substitute spare ribs in this recipe: They'll take the same amount of time to cook.

SERVES: 4
RECOMMENDED PELLETS:
Hickory, Oak

INGREDIENTS
2 racks baby back pork ribs (about 5 pounds total), trimmed
1/3 cup yellow mustard
1/2 cup apple juice (divided use), plus more if needed
1 tablespoon worcestershire sauce
Traeger Pork and Poultry Rub, or your favorite barbecue rub
1/2 Cup packed dark brown sugar
1/3 cup honey, warmed
Traeger BBQ Sauce, or your favorite barbecue sauce

DIRECTIONS
1. If your butcher has not already done so, remove the thin papery membrane from the bone-side of the ribs by working the tip of a butter knife or a screwdriver underneath the membrane over a middle bone. Use paper towels to get a firm grip, then tear the membrane off.

2. In a small bowl, combine the mustard, 1/4 cup of apple juice (reserve the rest), and the Worcestershire sauce. Spread thinly on both sides of the ribs; season with Traeger Pork and Poultry Rub.

3. When ready to cook, start the Traeger grill on Smoke with the lid open until the fire is established (4 to 5 minutes). Smoke the ribs, meat-side up, for 3 hours. Transfer the ribs to a rimmed baking sheet but leave the grill on. Set the temperature to 225 degrees F.

4. Tear off four long sheets of heavy duty aluminum foil. Top with a rack of ribs; pull up the sides to keep the liquid enclosed. Sprinkle half the brown sugar on the rack, then top with half the honey and half of the remaining apple juice. (Use a bit more apple juice if you want.) Lay another piece of foil on top and tightly crimp the edges so there's no leakage. Repeat with the remaining rack of ribs.

5. Return the foiled ribs to the grill and cook for an additional 2 hours. Carefully remove the foil from the ribs—watch out for hot steam—and brush the ribs on both sides with Traeger BBQ Sauce. Discard the foil. Arrange the ribs directly on the grill grate and continue to grill until the sauce "tightens", 30 minutes to 1 hour more. Let the ribs rest for a few minutes before serving.

MEMPHIS-STYLE BABY BACK RIBS

They like their ribs saucy and cooked low and slow in Kansas City and other places, but not in Memphis: There, the ribs are grilled directly over the heat, are seasoned after grilling, and are served sans barbecue sauce. Cooking time on these baby backs is only 2 to 3 hours—half the time of conventionally barbecued ribs—making them a good choice for busy days or nights.

SERVES: 4
RECOMMENDED PELLETS:
Hickory, Oak

INGREDIENTS

2 racks baby back pork ribs (about 5 pounds total), trimmed

Traeger Pork and Poultry Rub, or your favorite barbecue rub

2 Cups apple juice in a loaf pan or pie plate, plus more if needed

DIRECTIONS

1. If your butcher has not already done so, remove the thin papery membrane from the Hickory, Oak bone-side of the ribs by working the tip of a butter knife or a screwdriver underneath the membrane over a middle bone. Use paper towels to get a firm grip, then tear the membrane off.

2. When ready to cook, start the Traeger grill on Smoke with the lid open until the fire is established (4 to 5 minutes). Set the temperature to 325 degrees F and preheat, lid closed, for 10 to 15 minutes. Put the apple juice in a corner of the grill grate.

3. Arrange the ribs on the grill grate, meat- side up. Cook for 2 hours. Check the ribs. They should be nicely browned and tear apart easily in your fingers.

4. If they're not done to your liking, return them to the grill, checking them every 30 minutes. Replenish the apple juice if needed.

5. When the ribs are done, transfer them toa cutting board and season them with Traeger Pork and Poultry Rub. Let them rest for a
few minutes before cutting into half slabs or individual ribs.

PORK LOIN ROAST WITH SAUERKRAUT AND APPLES

Though traditional in many households for New Year's Day, pork loin roast is an economical choice any time of the year. For one thing, there's almost no waste; and for another, it's often on sale. If you can, try to find the plastic bags of sauerkraut often sold in the meat department or refrigerated section of supermarkets. Feel free, though, to substitute canned sauerkraut.

SERVES: 8
RECOMMENDED PELLETS:
Apple

INGREDIENTS
1-pound bag of refrigerated sauerkraut
2 cooking apples (such as granny smith), cored and chopped
1/3 cup brown sugar
1 pork loin roast, 2 to 2-1/2 pounds
Traeger Sweet Rub, or salt and pepper

DIRECTIONS
1. Spread the sauerkraut and apple pieces in the bottom of a 9- by 13-inch glass baking dish. Sprinkle evenly with the brown sugar. Season the pork roast with Traeger Sweet Rub and lay it on top of the sauerkraut-apple mixture, fat-side up.

2. When ready to cook, start the Traeger grill on Smoke with the lid open until the fire is established (4 to 5 minutes). Set the temperature to 350 degrees F.

3. Roast the pork for 1 to 1-1/2 hours, or until the internal temperature on an instant-read meat thermometer reads 160 degrees F. Transfer the meat to a cutting board and let rest. Meanwhile, stir the sauerkraut-apple mixture and arrange it on a platter. Slice the pork roast and shingle the slices on top of the sauerkraut and apples. Serve immediately.

BARBECUED PORK SHOULDER STEAKS

Pork shoulder steaks—also called blade steaks—are often a value at the meat counter. If you buy steaks that are thinner than one inch, make shallow vertical cuts in the fat around the edge of the steaks before cooking to discourage them from curling.

SERVES: 4
RECOMMENDED PELLETS:
Apple

INGREDIENTS
4 pork shoulder steaks, 1- to 1-1/4-inch thick
Traeger Pork and Poultry Rub, or your favorite rub
1 Cup Traeger Honey- Bourbon Barbecue Sauce, or your favorite barbecue sauce

DIRECTIONS
1. Season the pork steaks with the Traeger Pork and Poultry Rub.

2. When ready to cook, start the Traeger grill on Smoke with the lid open until the fire is established (4 to 5 minutes).

3. Arrange the steaks on the grill grate. Smoke for 1 hour.

4. Set the temperature to 325 degrees F and preheat, lid closed, for 10 to 15 minutes.

5. Grill the steaks for 35 to 40 minutes, or until they reach 160 degrees F on an instant- read meat thermometer. The last 15 minutes, brush each steak on both sides with the Traeger Honey-Bourbon Barbecue Sauce. Let the steaks rest for 3 minutes before serving.

STUFFED PORK CHOPS

They seldom appear on American tables these days, but stuffed pork chops deserve a comeback: tender, succulent pork chops with a savory dressing that gets deliciously crunchy on the outside. Baked apples, put on the Traeger when you start the chops, make a fine dessert.

SERVES: 4
RECOMMENDED PELLETS:
Apple

INGREDIENTS
4 thick-cut (1-inch) pork loin chops, preferably with pockets cut in each
2 cups herb-seasoned or cornbread stuffing mix, such as pepperidge farm
Traeger pork and poultry rub, or salt and freshly ground black pepper

DIRECTIONS
1. If your butcher has not already done so, cut a deep pocket in the side of each chop with a small sharp knife, cutting toward the bone, but not all the way through.

2. Prepare the stuffing mix according to the package directions, adding your own touches if desired (chopped onion or celery, finely diced apple, or browned sausage).

Generously stuff each pork chop pocket with the mixture. Season both sides of the chops with Traeger Pork and Poultry Rub.

3. When ready to cook, start the Traeger grill on Smoke with the lid open until the fire is established (4 to 5 minutes). Set the

temperature to 325 degrees F and preheat, lid closed, for 10 to 15 minutes.

4. Arrange the chops directly on the grill grate. Bake for 45 to 50 minutes, or until the pork is cooked (160 degrees F on an instant- read meat thermometer). There is no need to turn the chops. Let the pork rest for 2 to

3 minutes before transferring to a platter or plates.

HONEY-MUSTARD PORK TENDERLOIN

Lean pork tenderloin can be infamously dry—but not when coated with a savory mixture of mustard, honey, and mayonnaise, and cooked on a Traeger. Use fresh herbs if you have them. Accompany the pork with roasted or mashed potatoes and a green vegetable.

SERVES: 4
RECOMMENDED PELLETS:
Apple

INGREDIENTS
1/4 cup coarse-grain or Dijon-style mustard
2 tablespoons honey
2 tablespoons mayonnaise, such as Hellmann's
1 tablespoon chopped fresh parsley, rosemary, or tarragon, or 1-1/2 teaspoons dried
1-1/2 teaspoons Traeger Pork and Poultry Rub
2 pork tenderloins, each 12 to 14 ounces, silverskin trimmed

DIRECTIONS
1. In a small bowl, combine the mustard, honey, mayonnaise, parsley, and Traeger Pork and Poultry Rub; stir to mix. Lay the pork tenderloins in a flat baking dish. Pour the mustard-honey mixture over the tenderloins, turning to coat all sides. (If not cooking immediately, cover with plastic wrap and refrigerate.)

2. When ready to cook, start the Traeger grill on Smoke with the lid open until the fire is established (4 to 5 minutes). Set the
temperature to 325 degrees F and preheat, lid closed, for 10 to 15 minutes.

3. Lift the tenderloins out of the mustard- honey mixture and arrange on a diagonal on the grill grate. (Discard the remaining mustard-honey mixture.) Grill for 30 to 40 minutes, or until the pork reaches 160 degrees F on an instant-read meat thermometer. Transfer to a cutting board and let rest for 3 minutes. Slice into 3/4-inch slices and serve.

COUNTRY-STYLE BONELESS PORK RIBS

Country-style pork ribs come from the rib end of the sirloin and are very meaty, sometimes weighing nearly a half pound each. Fruit-based barbecue sauces pair beautifully with them.

SERVES: 4
RECOMMENDED PELLETS:
Apple, Cherry

INGREDIENTS
8 boneless country-style pork ribs
Traeger Pork and Poultry Rub, or your favorite barbecue rub
1 cup traeger apricot barbecue sauce, or your favorite fruit-based barbecue sauce

DIRECTIONS
1. Season the pork ribs on all sides with the Traeger Pork and Poultry Rub.

2. When ready to cook, start the Traeger grill on Smoke with the lid open until the fire is established (4 to 5 minutes).

3. Arrange the pork ribs directly on the grill grate and smoke for 1 hour. Increase the temperature to 250 degrees F. Continue cooking for 1-1/2 hour to 2 hours, or until the ribs are tender and have reached 155 degrees F on an instant-read meat thermometer. Using a basting brush, apply the Traeger Apricot Barbecue Sauce to the ribs, turning with tongs to reach all sides. Let them cook for 10 to 15 minutes more. Let the ribs rest for 3 minutes before serving.

PULLED PORK

Pulled pork is a project for a lazy day. You just can't rush it. The pork shoulder will take about 1-1/2 to 2 hours per pound to cook to perfection (190 degrees F), so start it early in the day if you want to serve it for dinner. A puckery vinegar-based sauce replaces barbecue sauce in Eastern North Carolina, where pulled pork is a religion. To make a Carolina-inspired sauce, combine 2 cups of vinegar (white, apple cider, or a combination of both) with 1 tablespoon each of brown sugar, salt, black pepper, and hot sauce in a canning jar. Add 2 teaspoons of crushed red pepper and let it sit for several hours before serving. This stuff is hot, but plays off the richness of the pork.

SERVES: 10
RECOMMENDED PELLET:
Apple, Hickory

INGREDIENTS

1 bone-in pork shoulder roast (also called Boston butt), about 5 pounds, outside fat trimmed to about 1/8-inch

Traeger Pork and Poultry Rub

2 cups apple juice in a food-safe spray bottle (optional)

traeger regular barbecue sauce

10 hamburger buns

DIRECTIONS

1. Generously season all sides of the pork roast with the rub.

2. When ready to cook, start the Traeger grill on Smoke with the lid open until the fire is established (4 to 5 minutes). Set the temperature to 225 degrees F and preheat, lid closed, for 10 to 15 minutes.

3. Put the roast on the grill grate, fat-side up, and cook for 3 hours, spraying with apple juice every hour after the first hour, if desired. Transfer to a disposable aluminum foil pan large enough to hold the meat, and roast for 5 or 6 additional hours, or until an instant-read meat thermometer inserted in the thickest part, but not touching bone, registers 190 degrees F. If the pork starts to brown too much, cover it loosely with aluminum foil.

4. Carefully transfer the pork shoulder to a cutting board and cover loosely with aluminum foil. Let it rest for 30 minutes.

Alternatively, you can wrap it tightly in foil and "hold" it in an insulated cooler for up to an hour. Pour the juices from the bottom of the aluminum foil pan into a gravy separator.

5. While the pork is still hot, pull it into chunks using forks or your hands (preferably protected from the heat with lined, heavy-duty rubber gloves). Discard the bone and any lumps of fat or connective tissue. Pull each chunk into shreds, and transfer to a large mixing bowl. Season with additional rub, if desired, and moisten with the reserved drippings (discard any fat that has floated to the top of the drippings). Add barbecue sauce, if desired, and mix well. Or serve the barbecue sauce on the side.

6. Pile the pork mixture on the hamburger buns and serve with coleslaw,if desired.

BAKED HAM WITH APRICOT-HORSERADISH GLAZE

Fully cooked hams, such as the one called for in this recipe, do not have to be heated to 160 degrees F like a raw product. In fact, you can serve them cold.

SERVES: 12-15
RECOMMENDED PELLETS:
Apple, Cherry

INGREDIENTS
1 whole bone-in ham (fully cooked), 12 to 15 pounds
13.1-ounce bottle Traeger Apricot Barbecue Sauce, or your favorite fruit-based barbecue sauce
1/4 cup prepared horseradish, or more to taste
2 tablespoons Dijon- style mustard

DIRECTIONS
1. If the ham still has a layer of fat and skin on it, trim the skin off, leaving about 1/4-INCh of fat on the meat. Line a large roasting pan with aluminum foil, allowing it to overhang the sides. (This will make clean-up easier.) Put the ham in the roaster.

2. In a saucepan, combine the Traeger Apricot Barbecue Sauce, the horseradish, and the mustard. Warm gently when the ham is nearly done.

3. When ready to cook, start the Traeger grill on Smoke with the lid open until the fire is established (4 to 5 minutes). Set the

temperature to 325 degrees F and preheat, lid closed, for 10 to 15 minutes.

4. Put the roaster with the ham on the grill grate and bake for 2-1/2 hours, or until the internal temperature of the ham is 135 degrees F when read on an instant-read meat thermometer. Brush the apricot-horseradish glaze over the outside of the ham. Continue to bake for an hour more. Transfer the ham to a cutting board and tent with aluminum foil. Allow it to rest for 20 minutes before carving and serving with the remaining apricot- horseradish glaze, preferably warmed on the grill or stovetop.

SMOKY CEDAR-PORK BURGERS

Bored with traditional beef burgers? Ground pork, seasoned with barbecue rub and barbecue sauce, is a nice change. Coleslaw makes a terrific accompaniment.

RECOMMENDED PELLET:
Hickory, Oak

INGREDIENTS
2 pounds ground pork, cold
1 cup grated cheddar cheese
2 tablespoons Traeger Regular Barbecue Sauce, or your favorite barbecue sauce, plus more for serving
2 tablespoons grated onion (optional)

1 tablespoon traeger pork and poultry shake, or your favorite barbecue rub, or more to taste
4 hamburger buns, for serving
Your favorite condiments (sliced onions, pickles, tomatoes, etc.)

DIRECTIONS

1. Put the pork, cheese, onion, if using, Traeger Regular Barbecue Sauce, and Traeger Pork and Poultry Rub in a mixing bowl. Run cold water over your hands, and use them to mix the meat, cheese, and seasonings. Rewet your hands if necessary. Form the meat mixture into 4 equal patties, and use your thumbs to form a large shallow depression on one side of each patty. (This will keep the burgers from bulging in the middle when grilled.)

2. When ready to cook, start the Traeger grill on Smoke with the lid open until the fire is established (4 to 5 minutes).

3. Arrange the burgers, depression-side down, on the grill grate and smoke for 30 minutes. Increase the temperature to 300 degrees F. Grill the burgers until an instant- read meat thermometer reads 160 degrees F, about 45 minutes. Turn the burgers halfway through the grilling time. Let rest for 2 to 3 minutes before serving to let the juices redistribute themselves. Serve on buns with additional Traeger Regular Barbecue Sauce and/or your favorite condiments.

TERIYAKI PORK AND PINEAPPLE SKEWERS

Sometimes, pork sirloin is sold in supermarkets already cubed and accompanied by wooden skewers. Usually, it is labeled "city chicken," a name it picked up during the Great Depression when pork was less expensive than chicken.

SERVES: 2-3
RECOMMENDED PELLETS:
Hickory, Oak

INGREDIENTS
1 pound pork sirloin cubes, each about 1- inch by 1-inch and 1/2- inch thick (18 pieces)
2 to 3 slices fresh pineapple, cored and cut into bite-size chunks
1 cup traeger carne asada marinade, or your favorite teriyaki marinade
6 large scallions (green onions), trimmed, pale and light green parts cut into 1-inch lengths
6 6- to 8-inch wooden skewers

DIRECTIONS
1. Thread a pork cube through the thin side on a skewer, followed by a chunk of pineapple and a piece of green onion; repeat the sequence twice to complete a skewer (three cubes of pork per skewer). Repeat with the other five skewers. Transfer the skewers to a glass pan or pie plate and pour the marinade over them, turning to coat on all sides. Cover with plastic wrap and refrigerate for 1 to 3 hours.

2. When ready to cook, start the Traeger grill on Smoke with the lid open until the fire is established (4 to 5 minutes). Set the temperature to 450 degrees F (High) and preheat, lid closed, for 10 to 15 minutes.

3. Drain the skewers, discarding the marinade. Arrange the skewers on the grill grate and grill, turning once, for 10 minutes, or until the pork is cooked through. Transfer the skewers to a platter or plates and serve immediately.

BRATS IN A BATH

This is a perfect recipe for tailgating or a game day party at home as the brats will stay hot for a long time in their "bath". If desired, you can smoke the brats before finishing them over higher heat.

SERVES: 5
RECOMMENDED PELLET:
Hickory, Oak, Pecan

DIRECTIONS
3 to 4 12-ounce cans of beer (dark or light)
2 large onions, peeled and sliced into rings
2 tablespoons butter, plus extra for buttering the buns
10 brats, uncooked
10 brat or hoagie buns
Mustard for serving

DIRECTIONS

1. Pour the beer into a saucepan. Add the onions and 2 tablespoons of butter. Bring to a simmer on the stovetop.

2. When ready to cook, start the Traeger grill on Smoke with the lid open until the fire is established (4 to 5 minutes). Set the temperature to 350 degrees F and preheat, lid closed, for 10 to 15 minutes.

3. Put a deep disposable aluminum foil pan on one side of the Traeger. Carefully pour the beer and onions from the saucepan into the pan on the grill. Arrange the brats on the other side of the grill grate. Grill the brats until cooked through, turning frequently with tongs, about 20 to 25 minutes. Transfer the brats to the beer bath and cover the pan tightly with aluminum foil. Let the brats simmer in the bath until the onions are tender, 45 minutes to an hour.

4. Butter the cut sides of the buns and toast on the grill. To serve, lift a brat out of the bath and put it on a bun. Top it with onions and mustard, if desired.

ITALIAN MILK-BRAISED PORK TENDERLOIN

While pork braised in milk is well-known in Italy, it is less common here. It is a simple but delicious preparation; the pork braises slowly in milk infused with fresh chopped rosemary and sage (use dried herbs if you must) and garlic. Don't be concerned if the milk curdles somewhat: It's supposed to.

Just break up the curds with a small whisk as directed below.

SERVES: 4-6
RECOMMENDED PELLETS:
Apple

INGREDIENTS
2 pork tenderloins, each about 1 pound
2 tablespoons extra- virgin olive oil (divided use)
2 tablespoons chopped fresh rosemary, or 2 teaspoons dried
2 tablespoons chopped fresh sage, or 2 teaspoons dried
Salt and freshly ground black pepper
2 cups whole milk, or half and half
1-1/2 teaspoons worcestershire sauce
2 cloves garlic, smashed
1 bay leaf

DIRECTIONS
1. Trim the pork tenderloins of any extra fat or silverskin. Rub the meat with a tablespoon of olive oil, then with the rosemary and sage. Season the tenderloins with salt and pepper.

2. On the stovetop, heat an ovenproof skillet over medium-high heat. Add the remaining tablespoon of olive oil to the skillet. Add the tenderloins and brown well on all sides, turning with tongs. Pour in the milk and add the Worcestershire sauce, garlic and bay leaf. Bring to a simmer.

3. When ready to cook, start the Traeger grill on Smoke with the lid open until the fire is established (4 to 5 minutes). Set the temperature to 325 degrees F and preheat, lid closed, for 10 to 15 minutes.

4. Carefully transfer the skillet with the pork and milk to the grill grate. (If you do not own an ovenproof skillet, simply transfer the pork and milk mixture to an baking dish and put that on the grill grate.) Braise for 1 hour, or until the pork is very tender and the milk has partially evaporated. (The internal temperature of the pork should be 160 degrees F.) Slice the pork into medallions and arrange on a platter. Remove the garlic
cloves and bay leaf from the milk mixture and discard. Whisk, then taste for seasoning, adding more salt and pepper if desired.
Pour the sauce over the pork and serve immediately.

TRAEGER POULTRY RECIPES

POULTRY TIPS

- Chicken should always be cooked to an internal temperature of 165 degrees F to kill food-borne pathogens like salmonella.
- Wash anything that has come in contact with raw poultry thoroughly with hot soapy water (hands, cutting boards, knives, platters, etc.) before reusing.
- Lightly smoke peeled, hard-cooked eggs on the Traeger for an interesting twist on deviled eggs or egg salad. (Smoke for about 30 minutes. Longer, and the outside of the egg membrane will toughen.)
- Whole chickens are usually less expensive than chicken parts. Learn how to break down whole birds to save money.
- Brine poultry before cooking for extra moistness and flavor. Mix 1/4 cup salt and 2 tablespoons of sugar with a quart of cold water; stir until the salt and sugar crystals dissolve. Submerge the poultry, then cover and refrigerate. Brine whole chickens or

turkeys overnight; brine breasts, thighs, and legs for 2 to 4 hours. Rinse, then dry thoroughly before proceeding with the recipe.

- Put aromatics such as onions, carrots, celery, herbs, or cut-up lemons or oranges in the cavity of a roasting bird for extra flavor.
- For better browning, rub the outside of the bird with melted butter or olive or vegetable oil before seasoning.
- Mix dried herbs or chopped fresh herbs and seasonings into softened butter, then refrigerate or freeze. Tuck it under the skin of roasting chickens to add richness, moistness, and flavor.

BASIC TRAEGER CHICKEN BREAST

Boneless, skinless chicken breasts are nothing if not versatile. On a few minutes' notice, you can fix a fine meal for company or family. You will be amazed by how moist the breasts are when grilled on a Traeger. Make extras to have on hand for salads, fajitas, nachos, sandwiches, etc.

SERVES: 6-8

RECOMMENDED PELLETS:
Alder, Pecan, Oak

INGREDIENTS
8 boneless, skinless chicken breasts, each about 6 ounces after tenders are removed (see Note below)
Traeger Pork and Poultry Rub, or salt and pepper, or your favorite seasoning blend

DIRECTIONS
1. Season each chicken breast on both sides with Traeger Pork and Poultry Rub.

2. When ready to cook, start the Traeger grill on Smoke with the lid open until the fire is established (4 to 5 minutes). Set the temperature to 350 degrees F and preheat, lid closed, for 10 to 15 minutes.

3. Arrange the chicken breasts on the grill grate and cook, turning once halfway through the cooking time, for 25 to 30 minutes, or until the internal temperature, when read on an instant-read meat thermometer, is 170 degrees F. Remove to a platter or plates and let rest for 2 minutes before serving.

Note: The small flap of meat on the underside of a chicken breast is called the tender. Oftentimes, the butcher has already removed it. The breast will grill more evenly and look more attractive if you remove the tender and grill it separately.

BRINED CHICKEN BREASTS WITH MANDARIN GLAZE

Perhaps you've heard of "brining," but have never tried it. In its simplest form, brining means soaking food in salty water for 30 minutes to several hours. It makes a noticeable difference in flavor, texture, and juiciness—especially in poultry. This particular dish is great when served with white rice.

SERVES: 6-8
RECOMMENDED PELLETS:
Apple, Cherry

INGREDIENTS
2 quarts cold water
1/2 cup kosher salt, or 1/4 cup if using table salt
1/4 cup brown sugar
1/2 cup soy sauce
8 boneless, skinless chicken breasts, each about 6 ounces after tenders are removed (see note below)
Traeger mandarin glaze, or chinese sweet chili sauce or sweet and sour sauce
2 scallions (green onions), trimmed and very thinly sliced, for garnish (optional)

DIRECTIONS
1. Make the brine: Pour the water, salt, brown sugar, and soy sauce into a large mixing bowl and stir until the sugar and salt dissolve. Submerge the chicken breasts in the brine, cover, and refrigerate for 2 to 4 hours (no longer, please). Drain the chicken and pat dry on paper towels. Discard the brine.

2. When ready to cook, start the Traeger grill on Smoke with the lid open until the fire is established (4 to 5 minutes). Set the
temperature to 350 degrees F and preheat, lid closed, for 10 to 15 minutes.

3. Arrange the chicken breasts on the grill grate and cook, turning once halfway through the cooking time, for 25 to 30 minutes, or until the internal temperature, when read on an instant-read meat thermometer is 170 degrees F. Brush the chicken breasts with the Traeger Mandarin Glaze during the last few minutes of cooking. Remove to a platter or plates and sprinkle the onions over the chicken breasts, if desired.

Note: The small flap of meat on the underside of a chicken breast is called the tender. Oftentimes, the butcher has already removed it. The breast will grill more evenly and look more attractive if you remove the tender and grill it separately.

BARBECUED CHICKEN THIGHS

Thighs are not only one of the tastiest parts of the chicken, but they are often a bargain at the meat counter. A short dip in ranch-style dressing ensures they'll be moist when you bring them to the table. Feel free to substitute another dressing—Italian, Caesar, or vinaigrette—if that's what you have in your pantry.

SERVES: 4
RECOMMENDED PELLETS:
Hickory, Oak, Pecan

INGREDIENTS
1-1/2 pounds chicken thighs, bone-in, skin-on (see Note below)
Traeger Chicken Rub, or your favorite poultry rub
1 Cup ranch-style dressing
1/2 teaspoon coarsely ground black pepper

DIRECTIONS
1. Trim the chicken thighs of any excess fat. Season with the Traeger Chicken Rub.

2. In a large mixing bowl, combine the ranch dressing and pepper, and stir to combine. Add the chicken thighs and toss gently with your hands to coat the thighs thoroughly. Cover and refrigerate for 1 to 2 hours, if desired, or cook immediately.

3. When ready to cook, start the Traeger grill on Smoke with the lid open until the fire is established (4 to 5 minutes). Set the temperature to 350 degrees F and preheat, lid closed, for 10 to 15 minutes.

4. Lift the chicken from the marinade (discard any left in the bowl). Arrange the chicken thighs, skin-side down, on the grill grate.
Grill for 40 to 45 minutes, or until the chicken reaches 170 degrees F on an instant-read meat thermometer. Do not turn the chicken while it is cooking. Transfer the chicken to a platter or plates. Let rest for 2 minutes before serving.

Note: If you prefer boneless skinless chicken thighs, shorten the cooking time to 30 minutes.

NO FUSS ROASTED CHICKEN

Nothing complicated here. Just oil the bird, season it, and let your Traeger work its magic. In less than an hour and a half, you'll have crisp skin and succulent meat with a hint of wood smoke. Do two chickens, and you'll have leftovers to look forward to.

SERVES: 4
RECOMMMENDED PELLETS:
Apple, Pecan

INGREDIENTS
One chicken, 4 to 5 pounds
Extra-virgin olive oil or vegetable oil
Traeger Chicken Rub, your favorite rub, or salt and pepper

DIRECTIONS
1. Remove any giblets from the cavity of the chicken, as well as any excess fat. Wash the chicken inside and out with cold running water. Dry thoroughly with paper towels.

2. Oil the outside of the bird and season with the Traeger Chicken Rub. Tuck the chicken wings behind the back. Tie the legs together with butcher's string. (This gives you a moister bird and a more attractive presentation.)

3. When ready to cook, start the Traeger grill on Smoke with the lid open until the fire is established (4 to 5 minutes). Set the temperature to 450 degrees F (High) and preheat, lid closed, for 10 to 15 minutes.

4. Place the chicken on the grill grate, breast- side up, and close the lid. Roast the chicken until an instant-read meat thermometer inserted into the thickest part of a thigh registers a temperature of 165 degrees F, 70 to 90 minutes. Remove the chicken to a platter and allow it to rest for 5 minutes. Untie the legs and carve.

GREEK-STYLE CHICKEN WITH GARLIC AND LEMON

Small potatoes tossed in olive oil and salt and pepper and then roasted alongside the chicken make an easy and delicious side dish. A green salad rounds out the meal.

SERVES: 8
RECOMMENDED PELLETS:
Oak, Pecan, Hickory

INGREDIENTS
2 roasting chickens (3- 1/2 to 4 pounds each), each cut into 8 pieces
2 lemons, cut into quarters through the stem ends
1/3 cup extra-virgin olive oil
4 cloves garlic, finely minced
1-1/2 tablespoons dried oregano
Traeger chicken rub or pork and poultry shake, or salt and coarsely ground black pepper
1 cup chicken broth

DIRECTIONS
1. Arrange the chicken pieces in a single layer in a large roasting pan (if desired, use a disposable aluminum foil roasting pan). Squeeze the juice from each piece of lemon over the chicken, catching any seeds in your fingers. Tuck the lemon rinds in with the chicken. Drizzle the olive oil over all.

Sprinkle the garlic over the chicken. Dust the chicken with the dried oregano, and season it generously with one of the two suggested Traeger rubs, or salt and black pepper. Pour the chicken broth into the pan.

2. When ready to cook, start the Traeger grill on Smoke with the lid open until the fire is established (4 to 5 minutes). Set the temperature to 350 degrees F and preheat, lid closed, for 10 to 15 minutes.

3. Roast the chicken for an hour, or until the juices run clear or the internal temperature reaches 165 degrees F on an instant-read meat thermometer. Transfer to a platter or plates and spoon some of the juices on top. Let rest for 3 minutes before serving.

BARBECUED CHICKEN QUARTERS

Let's face it: the barbecued chicken of our youth often promised more than it delivered. Charred on the outside and raw on the inside, it tested the mettle of the most dedicated grill masters of the day. In their defense, they were generally working with grills that were nothing more than shallow pans with a grill grate, grills that were designed for direct grilling only. Flare-ups were a force to be reckoned with. Not so with a Traeger, which grills indirectly. Your chicken need not fear the flame.

SERVES: 4-6
RECOMMENDED PELLETS:
Apple, Cherry, Pecan

INGREDIENTS
6 leg and thigh quarters, about 5 to 6 pounds
Vegetable oil or extra- virgin olive oil
Traeger chicken rub, or your favorite all-purpose barbecue rub
2 cups traeger regular barbecue sauce, or your favorite barbecue sauce

DIRECTIONS
1. Wash the chicken under cold running water and pat dry with paper towels.

2. Oil each quarter, then season with Traeger Chicken Rub.

3. When ready to cook, start the Traeger grill on Smoke with the lid open until the fire is established (4 to 5 minutes). Set the temperature to 350 degrees F and preheat, lid closed, for 10 to 15 minutes.

4. Arrange the chicken quarters on the grill grate, skin-side up. Roast for 1 to 1-1/2 hours, or until the internal temperature (insert the probe of an instant-read meat thermometer into the thickest part of the thigh, but not touching bone) reads 165 degrees F. Using a basting brush, apply barbecue sauce to both sides of the chicken the last 15 minutes of cooking, turning once. (If you apply the sauce too early, the sugars in the sauce could caramelize and scorch.) Let rest for 5 minutes, then serve.

BUFFALO CHICKEN WRAPS

All the flavors of that American classic—Buffalo wings—without the bones and in an easy-to-eat form! Chicken tenders are often a bargain at the supermarket. But feel free to substitute boneless skinless chicken breasts cut lengthwise into one-inch strips.

SERVES: 4
RECOMMENDED PELLETS:
Hickory, Oak

INGREDIENTS
1-1/4 pounds chicken tenders
Traeger cajun shake or pork and poultry shake, or salt and freshly ground black pepper
3 tablespoons butter
1/2 cup hot sauce, such as frank's redhot
1-1/2 cups shredded lettuce
1 cup diced celery
1/2 cup prepared blue cheese or ranch dressing
4 10-inch flour tortillas

DIRECTIONS
1. Season the chicken tenders on all sides with the Traeger Cajun Shake or Pork and Poultry Shake.

2. When ready to cook, start the Traeger grill on Smoke with the lid open until the fire is established (4 to 5 minutes). Set the
temperature to 350 degrees F and preheat, lid closed, for 10 to 15 minutes.

3. Arrange the chicken tenders on the grill grate. Cook for 20 minutes, or until the chicken is no longer pink inside. While the chicken is cooking, melt the butter in a saucepan. Add the hot sauce and stir to combine. Using tongs, transfer the cooked chicken tenders to the hot sauce mixture, turning to coat.

4. If desired, briefly warm the tortillas on the grill. (They are easier to handle when warm.) Lay the tortillas on a flat work surface. Using tongs, lift the chicken tenders from the sauce and arrange on the tortillas. Top with the lettuce and celery. Drizzle with the blue cheese or ranch dressing, and roll up, burrito-style. Serve immediately.

BASIC BEER CAN CHICKEN

Beer can chicken is now a staple in North American backyards. And for good reason: it's super-moist. But the truth is, you don't have to use beer. Canned fruit juice, tea, soda pop, etc., work just as well. Make sure your model of Traeger grill has enough clearance to accommodate your upright chicken before starting this recipe. If not, substitute Cornish game hens for chicken (one per diner) and replace the beer cans with 6-ounce fruit or vegetable juice cans. Cooking time will be slightly less—about one hour total.

SERVE: 5
RECOMMENDED PELLET:
Hickory, Alder, Oak, Pecan

INGREDIENTS
3-1/2 to 4 pound chicken, giblets removed
2 tablespoons vegetable oil
Traeger chicken rub or pork or poultry rub, or your favorite barbecue rub
12-ounce can of beer

DIRECTIONS
1. Remove any extra fat from the body and neck cavities. Rinse the chicken, inside and out, with cold running water. Drain and blot dry with paper towels. Transfer the chicken to a baking pan. Oil the outside of the chicken. Season the chicken with the Traeger Chicken Rub, including the neck and body cavities. Fold the wing tips behind the chicken's back.

2. Open the beer and pour half into a glass. (What you do with the beer in the glass is up to you.) Using a "church key" can opener, make an additional hole or two in the top of the beer can. Set it in the baking pan. This keeps the rub from going everywhere and makes it easier to transport to the grill. Carefully ease the chicken onto the beer can so the can rests in the body cavity. Bring the legs of the chicken forward so they form a tripod with the beer can. Touch up any places where the rub was disturbed.

3. When ready to cook, start the Traeger grill on Smoke with the lid open until the fire is established (4 to 5 minutes). Set the temperature to 350 degrees F and preheat, lid closed, for 10 to 15 minutes.

4. Carefully transfer the chicken on its beer can to the grill grate, positioning it where the grill lid is highest. Cook the chicken until the skin is golden brown and the internal temperature inserted in the thickest part of the thigh reads 170 degrees F on an instant-read meat thermometer, about 1-1/4 to 1-1/2 hours. If the top of the chicken browns too quickly, cover it loosely with aluminum foil. Carefully transfer the chicken on its can to a platter or clean baking pan. Let the chicken rest for 5 minutes before carefully removing the beer can. Carve and serve.

CHEESY CHICKEN ENCHILADAS

This dish is a real crowd-pleaser, but only takes minutes to assemble if you have the cooked chicken on hand from a previous Traeger grill session. (Cooked turkey can stand in for the chicken.) Serve with rice, refried black beans, and shredded lettuce and radishes.

SERVES: 6
RECOMMENDED PELLETS:
Hickory, Oak, Mesquite

INGREDIENTS
6 cups shredded or cubed cooked chicken
3 cups grated mexican- blend cheese, or monterey jack or mild cheddar (12 ounces), divided use
1 cup sour cream or mexican crema

1 cup pitted sliced black olives

4-ounce can chopped green chiles

2 10-ounce cans green or red enchilada sauce (divided use)

12 8-inch flour tortillas

3 scallions (green onions), trimmed, white and green parts thinly sliced, for serving (optional)

Fresh cilantro leaves, chopped, for serving (optional)

DIRECTIONS

1. Make the filling: In a large mixing bowl, combine the cooked chicken and 2 Cups of the cheese. Stir in the sour cream, black olives, and green chiles and mix well.

2. Pour one can of the enchilada sauce into the bottom of a 13- by 9-inch baking dish. Spoon about 1/3 cup of the filling on the lower third of each tortilla and roll up. Transfer to the baking dish, long sides of the enchiladas touching. When you have assembled all of the tortillas, pour the second can of enchilada sauce over the tops, using a spoon or spatula to coat the outside of each tortilla with the sauce. Sprinkle the remaining cup of cheese down the center of the row of rolled tortillas. Cover the baking dish tightly with foil.

3. When ready to cook, start the Traeger grill on Smoke with the lid open until the fire is established (4 to 5 minutes). Set the temperature to 350 degrees F and preheat, lid closed, for 10 to 15 minutes.

4. Bake the enchiladas for 30 minutes. Then remove the foil, and bake for 15 more minutes, or until the enchiladas are hot and the cheese is melted. Garnish with sliced scallions and chopped fresh cilantro, if desired. Serve hot.

FIRST TIMER'S TURKEY

There's no need to stress about the turkey when you have Traeger on your team. It couldn't be easier. You can even avoid gravy-making by recruiting a talented gravy meister or buying a good-quality jarred gravy. While many people carve the turkey breast with their knife parallel to the breast bone, we've found it's better to remove the entire breast and then cut it crosswise. That way, everyone who loves white meat gets both meat and skin.

SERVE: 6
RECOMMENDED PELLETS:
Apple, Pecan

INGREDIENTS
1 turkey (thawed if previously frozen), 10 to 12 pounds
Extra-virgin olive oil or vegetable oil
Traeger Pork and Poultry Rub, or salt and freshly ground black pepper

You'll also need: a large sturdy roasting pan; butcher's string; an instant-read meat thermometer

DIRECTIONS

1. Remove the giblets from the body and neck cavities. (If your turkey came with a gravy packet, remove that, too.) Wash the turkey inside and out with cold running water and pat dry with paper towels. Inspect the bird for any remaining feathers, and remove these with kitchen tweezers.

2. Position the turkey in the roasting pan and brush it evenly with the oil. Season the skin with Traeger Pork and Poultry Rub. If your turkey came with a string sling for easy
removal from the pan once the bird is roasted, position it under the bird according to the package directions.

3. When ready to cook, start the Traeger grill on Smoke with the lid open until the fire is established (4 to 5 minutes). Set the temperature to 325 degrees F and preheat, lid closed, for 10 to 15 minutes.

4. Put the roasting pan with the turkey directly on the grill grate. Roast the turkey for 3 hours. Insert the probe from the meat thermometer in the thickest part of the thigh, but not touching bone: You're looking for a temperature of 165 degrees F. The turkey should also be beautifully browned with crisp skin. If the temperature is less than that, or if your turkey is not browned to your liking, let it roast for another 30 minutes, then check the temperature again. Repeat until the turkey is fully cooked.

5. When the turkey is done, carefully transfer it to a cutting board and let it rest for 20 minutes. Do not tent it with aluminum foil or the skin will lose its crispness.

6. Carve and serve.

SMOKED TURKEY LEGS

Amusement parks and fairs have given smoked turkey legs a cult-like following, with some people offering money online for a recipe that mimics the legs sold at Disneyland. The secret is to soak the legs in brine for 24 hours, then smoke them low and slow. The flavor is ham-like, and very addictive.

SERVES: 4
RECOMMENDED PELLETS:
Apple, Pecan

INGREDIENTS

1 gallon cold water
1 cup morton's tender quick®
1/4 cup brown sugar
6 allspice berries, crushed (optional)
6 whole black peppercorns
2 bay leaves, broken into pieces
6 whole cloves
2 teaspoons liquid smoke
6 turkey legs, each weighing about 1.5 pounds (see note below)

DIRECTIONS

1. In a large stockpot, combine one gallon of water, the rub, curing salt, brown sugar, allspice (if using), peppercorns, bay leaves, cloves, and liquid smoke. . Bring to a boil over high heat to dissolve the salt granules. Cool to room temperature, then refrigerate until thoroughly chilled. Add the turkey legs, making sure they're completely submerged in the brine. You can hold them down with a resealable bag filled with ice.

2. After 24 hours, drain the turkey legs and discard the brine. Rinse the brine off the legs with cold water, then dry thoroughly with paper towels. Brush off any clinging solid spices.

3. When ready to cook, start the Traeger grill on Smoke with the lid open until the fire is established (4 to 5 minutes). Set the temperature to 225 degrees F and preheat, lid closed, for 10 to 15 minutes.

4. Lay the turkey legs directly on the grill grate. Cook for 4 to 5 hours, or until the internal temperature reaches 165 degrees F on an instant-read meat thermometer. (Make sure the probe doesn't touch bone or you'll get a false reading.) The turkey legs should be deeply browned. Do not be alarmed if the meat under the skin is pinkish: That's a chemical reaction to the cure and the smoke called a "smoke ring". Serve immediately, or refrigerate.

Note: If you can't find these Flintstone- esque legs, you can substitute smaller ones. Reduce the cooking time accordingly.

TRAEGER LAMB RECIPES

LAMB TIPS

- Lamb blade or round-bone shoulder chops are often significantly less expensive than rib or loin chops.
- Buy grass-fed lamb when possible for the best texture and flavor.
- Marinate lamb overnight in bottled vinaigrette or a marinade of your own making.
- Lamb shanks are terrific when cooked low and slow on your Traeger in a savory liquid.

(Cover tightly and allow at least four hours for the shanks to become tender.)

- Butterflied boneless leg of lamb is a quick and easy meal for a weeknight. Oftentimes, it is rolled and secured with elastic netting. Simply remove the netting before marinating or seasoning the lamb, then lay flat on the grill grate.

- The richness of lamb can be balanced with acids such as wine, vinegar, or lemon juice.

RACK OF LAMB

Many recipes for rack of lamb call for it to be seared in hot oil before roasting. But there's no need: the seasoned lamb can go right into the Traeger. The term "frenched" (see below) refers to a chop—usually lamb or veal—that has had the rib bones scraped for a more attractive presentation on the plate.

SERVES: 4
RECOMMENDED PELLETS:
Apple, Cherry

INGREDIENTS
8-bone rack of lamb, 1-1/2 pounds, frenched and trimmed of excess fat (leave 1/4-INCh), at room temperature
Extra-virgin olive oil or vegetable oil
Traeger Prime Rib Rub or Beef Rub, or coarse salt and freshly ground black pepper

2 tablespoons fresh herbs, such as rosemary, parsley, or thyme, or two teaspoons dried

DIRECTIONS

1. Rub the rack of lamb with olive oil and season with Traeger Prime Rib Rub and the herbs.

2. When ready to cook, start the Traeger grill on Smoke with the lid open until the fire is established (4 to 5 minutes). Set the temperature to 400 degrees F and preheat, lid closed, for 10 to 15 minutes.

3. Place the lamb on the grill grate, rounded- side up. Roast for 30 minutes for medium rare (135 degrees F on an instant-read meat thermometer inserted into the center of the meat, but not touching bone), longer if you like your lamb less rare.

4. Transfer the lamb to a cutting board and let it rest for 5 minutes. Slice into 2-BONE sections.

ROAST BUTTERFLIED LEG OF LAMB

Butterflied boneless leg of lamb is often sold rolled into a roast-like shape and held together with netting. You can leave it in the netting if desired, but a rolled roast is best cooked at a lower temperature—325 degrees F for 10 to 12 minutes per pound, or until it reaches medium-rare. You can cook bone-in lamb the same way. The marinade below is also excellent on rack of lamb and lamb chops.

SERVES: 6
RECOMMENDED PELLETS:
Pecan, Cherry, Apple

INGREDIENTS
one lemon washed
1/4 cup red wine vinegar
4 cloves garlic, minced
2 tablespoons minced fresh rosemary leaves, or 2 teaspoons dried
2 teaspoons fresh thyme, minced, or 1 teaspoon dried
1 teaspoon salt
1 teaspoon freshly ground black pepper
1 cup extra-virgin olive oil
1 onion, sliced into rings
4- to 5-pound butterflied (boneless) leg of lamb

DIRECTIONS

1. Make the marinade: Cut the lemon into quarters and remove the seeds. Squeeze Pecan, Cherry, Apple the juice into a mixing bowl, reserving the lemon rinds. Add the red wine vinegar, garlic, rosemary, thyme, and salt and pepper and stir until the salt crystals dissolve. Whisk in the olive oil.

Remove any netting from the lamb. Put the lamb into a large resealable plastic bag. Pour in the marinade, and add the onion and the reserved lemon rinds. Massage the bag to distribute the marinade and herbs. Refrigerate for several hours, or overnight.

2. Remove the lamb from the marinade and pat dry with paper towels. Discard the marinade.

3. When ready to cook, start the Traeger grill on Smoke with the lid open until the fire is established (4 to 5 minutes). Set the temperature to 450 degrees F (High) and preheat, lid closed, for 10 to 15 minutes.

4. Arrange the lamb on the grill grate, fat- side down. Grill 10 to 15 minutes per side for medium-rare (135 degrees F on an instant- read meat thermometer), longer if you prefer your lamb more well done. Let rest for 5 minutes. Slice thinly across the grain, and serve.

GRILLED LAMB CHOPS WITH CHILI-MINT SAUCE

Small, succulent lamb chops are great candidates for "Traegering." They are best when served medium-rare.

SERVES: 4
RECOMMENDED PELLETS:
Alder, Cherry, Apple

INGREDIENTS
8 loin lamb chops, 3/4- inch thick (about 4 to 5 ounces each), or lamb rib chops
1/2 cup distilled white vinegar or white wine
1 teaspoon salt
1/2 teaspoon freshly ground black pepper
2 tablespoons grated or finely minced onion
1 tablespoon fresh mint, chopped
2 tablespoons extra- virgin olive oil
Traeger prime rib rub, or salt and pepper
1/2 cup mint jelly
1/4 cup traeger mandarin glaze sauce, or your favorite chinese sweet chili sauce

DIRECTIONS
1. Using a sharp knife, trim any excess fat off the lamb chops and transfer the chops to a large resealable plastic bag. In a small mixing bowl, combine the vinegar and salt and pepper and stir until the salt dissolves. Stir in the onion, mint, and olive oil. Pour over the lamb chops and refrigerate for 2 to 4 hours.

2. Drain the lamb chops and pat dry with paper towels. Season on both sides with the Traeger Prime Rib Rub, or salt and pepper.

3. When ready to cook, start the Traeger grill on Smoke with the lid open until the fire is established (4 to 5 minutes). Set the temperature to 450 degrees F (High) and preheat, lid closed, for 10 to 15 minutes.

4. Arrange the chops on the grill grate. Grill for 4 to 6 minutes per side for medium-rare (130 to 135 degrees F on an instant-read meat thermometer). Meanwhile, combine the mint jelly and the Traeger Mandarin Glaze Sauce in a small saucepan. Warm on the stovetop or grill until the jelly is melted, stirring occasionally. Serve with the lamb chops.

TRAEGER SEAFOOD RECIPES

GLAZED SALMON

A restaurant-caliber meal in around 30 minutes? It's possible with your Traeger. Especially if you have access to fresh wild-caught salmon, preferably from the Pacific. Lemon wedges and sprigs of fresh tarragon or dill will give your plates visual appeal.

SERVES: 4
RECOMMENDED PELLETS:
Alder, Pecan

INGREDIENTS
4 center-cut salmon fillets with skin on, each 6 to 8-ounces
Traeger salmon shake, or salt and freshly ground black pepper
1/2 cup mayonnaise, preferably hellmann's
2 tablespoons dijon- style mustard
1 tablespoon fresh lemon juice
1 tablespoon chopped fresh tarragon or dill, or 1 teaspoon dried

DIRECTIONS

1. Remove any pin bones in the salmon with kitchen tweezers or needle-nose pliers. Season the fillets with the Traeger Salmon Shake. Make the glaze: Combine the mayonnaise and mustard in a small bowl. Stir in the lemon juice and tarragon. Spread the flesh-side of the fillets with the glaze.

2. When ready to cook, start the Traeger grill on Smoke with the lid open until the fire is established (4 to 5 minutes). Set the temperature to 350 degrees F and preheat, lid closed, for 10 to 15 minutes.

3. Arrange the salmon fillets on the grill grate, skin-side down. Grill for 25 to 30 minutes, or until the salmon is opaque and flakes easily with a fork. Transfer to a platter or plates and serve immediately.

CEDAR-PLANKED SALMON WITH LEMON-DILL BUTTER

While this is an impressive dinner for company, it is easy enough for a busy weeknight supper. Any leftover Lemon-Dill Butter pairs beautifully with grilled shrimp.

SERVES: 4
RECOMMENDED PELLETS:
Maple, Apple

INGREDIENTS
1 lemon
8 tablespoons (1 stick) butter, at room temperature
2 tablespoons fresh dill, chopped
Traeger salmon shake, or salt and freshly ground black pepper
4 skinless salmon fillets, preferably center-cut (6- to 8-ounces each)
1 untreated cedar plank (approximately 16- by 8-inches), soaked in water to cover for 1 hour, then drained (see note below)

DIRECTIONS
1. Wash the lemon, and cut it in half through its equator. Slice one-half into thin slices with a sharp knife and reserve (discard stem end). Remove the yellow zest from the other half with a knife or vegetable peeler and finely mince, or use a zester. Squeeze the juice from the zested half, discarding any seeds.

2. Make the Lemon-Dill Butter: In a small mixing bowl, combine the butter with the lemon zest, 1 tablespoon of lemon juice, the dill, and 1-1/2 teaspoons Traeger Salmon Shake or 1 teaspoon of salt and 1/2 teaspoon freshly ground black pepper. Set aside or cover and refrigerate if not using immediately. (The Lemon-Dill Butter can also be frozen for up to 6 months.)

3. When ready to cook, start the Traeger grill on Smoke with the lid open until the fire is established (4 to 5 minutes). Put the cedar plank directly on the grill grate. Set the temperature to 350 degrees F and preheat, lid closed, for 20 minutes. (This is a longer preheat than usual because you want to get the plank hot.)

4. Remove any pin bones from the salmon fillets (you can feel the bones with your fingertips) with kitchen tweezers or needle-nosed pliers. Season the salmon fillets on both sides with Traeger Salmon Shake. Arrange the fillets on the plank, and top each fillet with a slice of lemon. Cook, lid closed, for 25 to 30 minutes, or until the salmon is opaque and flakes easily when pressed with a fork. Top each fillet with a pat of Lemon-Dill Butter. Carefully transfer the fillets to a platter or plates and serve immediately.

Note: A rimmed cookie sheet works well for soaking the plank. Keep it submerged by resting something heavy, like a dinner plate, on the plank.

BAKED COD

For an easy side dish, slice the tops off ripe tomatoes. Salt and pepper them, then top them with grated Parmesan or Romano cheese and dust with dried basil. Bake the tomatoes alongside the fish.

SERVES: 4
RECOMMENDED PELLETS:
Oak

INGREDIENTS
4 pieces cod loin (each about 8-ounces)
Juice of 1 lemon
1/2 cup (1 stick) butter, melted (divided use)
Traeger salmon shake, or salt and freshly ground black pepper
25 round buttery snack crackers, such as ritz, crushed into fine crumbs
1-1/2 teaspoons dried basil
Chopped fresh parsley for garnish (optional)

DIRECTIONS
1. Arrange the cod in a buttered 9- by 13-inch baking pan and drizzle it with the lemon juice and 1/4 cup of the melted butter. Season the fish with the Traeger Salmon Shake. Combine the cracker crumbs, the basil, and the remainder of the butter in a small bowl and stir to mix. Top the cod with the crumb mixture.

2. When ready to cook, start the Traeger grill on Smoke with the lid open until the fire is established (4 to 5 minutes). Set the temperature to 400 degrees F and preheat, lid closed, for 10 to 15 minutes.

3. Put the baking dish on the grill grate and bake for 20 minutes, or until the topping is golden brown and the fish flakes easily when pressed with a fork. Garnish with parsley, if desired.

CITRUS-GRILLED SWORDFISH

This is an easy way to prepare firm, mild-tasting fish like monkfish, Chilean sea bass, halibut, etc.

SERVES: 4
RECOMMENDED PELLETS:
Alder, Oak, Pecan

DIRECTIONS

1. Slice the grapefruit into eighths. (If using the oranges and lime, cut each fruit into quarters.) Rub each swordfish steak on both sides with olive oil. Season with Traeger Salmon Shake.

2. When ready to cook, start the Traeger grill on Smoke with the lid open until the fire is established (4 to 5 minutes). Set the temperature to 450 degrees F (High) and preheat, lid closed, for 10 to 15 minutes.

3. Arrange the swordfish steaks on the grill grate. Squeeze the citrus juice (from 2 to 3 wedges of grapefruit) over the top of the steaks. Grill for 6 to 8 minutes. Using a thin spatula, turn the steaks. Again, squeeze citrus juice over the top of the steaks. Finish cooking the steaks, 6 to 8 minutes more, or until the flesh is opaque and breaks into firm flakes when pressed with a fork. Finish with a final squeeze of citrus juice.

Note: Citrus fruits will yield more juice if you microwave them for 20 to 30 seconds first.

BAKED BEANS

Chopped barbecued pork or beef brisket leftover from a previous grill session is a great addition to these beans. If you like your beans on the spicy side, add a few shakes of hot sauce, or sauté a minced jalapeno pepper along with the bacon, onion, and bell pepper.

SERVES: 15-18
RECOMMENDED PELLETS:
Hickory, Oak, Mesquite

INGREDIENTS
10 slices meaty thick- sliced smoked bacon, cold, diced
1 large sweet onion, peeled and diced
1 red or green bell pepper, stemmed, cored, and diced
28-ounce cans pork and beans
1 cup traeger regular barbecue sauce, or your favorite barbecue sauce
1/2 cup packed brown sugar
1/4 cup apple cider vinegar
1/4 cup worcestershire sauce
3 tablespoons prepared mustard
1-1/2 teaspoons ground clove

DIRECTIONS

1. Put the diced bacon in a cold skillet. Turn the heat to medium-low, and cook until the bacon has rendered some of its fat. Add the onion and the bell pepper and sauté until the vegetables soften. Transfer to a large mixing bowl. Stir in the pork and beans, barbecue sauce, brown sugar, vinegar, Worcestershire sauce, mustard, and clove. Pour into a large baking pan.

2. When ready to cook, start the Traeger grill on Smoke with the lid open until the fire is established (4 to 5 minutes). Set the temperature to 300 degrees F and preheat, lid closed, for 10 to 15 minutes.

3. Cook the beans for 2-1/2 to 3 hours, or until the liquid in the beans is syrupy. (Don't let them dry out.) Let the beans sit for a few minutes before serving.

HALIBUT WITH MEDITERRANEAN RELISH

Pantry items can be turned into a delicious relish for swordfish or other firm- fleshed fish like tuna, monkfish, salmon, or swordfish.

SERVES: 4
RECOMMENDED PELLETS:
Pecan, Oak, or Hickory

INGREDIENTS
1/2 cup pitted green olives, chopped
1/2 cup pitted black olives, chopped
1/4 cup sun-dried tomatoes, drained of oil, and chopped
1/4 cup chopped onion
1 clove garlic, minced
1 tablespoon red wine vinegar or freshly squeezed lemon juice
3 tablespoons extra- virgin olive oil, plus more for brushing the fish
Coarse salt and freshly ground black pepper
6-ounce halibut steaks, each about 3/4- inch thick, or another firm-fleshed fish (see suggestions above)

DIRECTIONS
1. Make the relish: In a small mixing bowl, combine the green and black olives, sun-dried tomatoes, onion, garlic, red wine vinegar, and 3 tablespoons of olive oil—season with freshly ground black pepper.

2. Brush the halibut steaks with olive oil and season on both sides with salt and freshly ground black pepper.

3. When ready to cook, start the Traeger grill on Smoke with the lid open until the fire is established (4 to 5 minutes). Set the temperature to 400 degrees F and preheat, lid closed, for 10 to 15 minutes.

4. Bake the fish for 15 to 20 minutes, or until it is opaque and flakes easily when pressed with a fork. Transfer to a platter or plates and top each steak with the olive relish.

PEPPERED TUNA WITH FRESH TOMATO AND MOZZARELLA SALAD

Tuna, tomatoes, mozzarella, and olive oil evoke the island of Sicily, just under the sole of the Italian boot. Accompany with good crusty bread.

SERVES: 4
RECOMMENDED PELLETS:
Alder, Oak

INGREDIENTS
4 tuna steaks (about 1-inch thick, 6 to 8 ounces each)

1/2 cup extra-virgin olive oil
coarsely ground black pepper
coarse salt (kosher or sea)
1 tablespoon red wine vinegar, or more to taste
1 pint (2 cups) cherry tomatoes, washed and halved lengthwise
4 ounces mozzarella, preferably fresh, cut into bite-size pieces
6 leaves fresh basil, chopped, or 1 teaspoon, dried
lemon wedges, for serving

DIRECTIONS

1. Trim any skin or dark spots off the tuna, if necessary. Oil both sides of each steak.
Generously season with coarsely ground black pepper and salt to taste. In a small bowl, combine 1/2 teaspoon black pepper and 1/2 teaspoon salt with the vinegar and stir until the salt dissolves. Whisk in the remaining olive oil, and stir in the basil.
In a larger bowl, combine the tomatoes and mozzarella. Set aside.

2. When ready to cook, start the Traeger grill on Smoke with the lid open until the fire is established (4 to 5 minutes). Set the temperature to 450 degrees F (High) and preheat, lid closed, for 10 to 15 minutes.

3. Arrange the tuna steaks on the grill grate and grill, turning once, until the steaks are browned on the outside and the desired degree of doneness is reached, 3 to 4 minutes per side for rare—longer for tuna that is fully cooked (approximately 8 to 10 minutes per side). Rewhisk the dressing, pour over the tomatoes and mozzarella, and toss gently.

Transfer the tuna steaks to plates and divide the tomato and mozzarella salad between them. (Plate with the salad just to the side of the tuna.) Serve with lemon wedges for squeezing.

TRAEGER MACARONI AND CHEESE FOR A CROWD

Nothing fancy here, but this is a supremely satisfying macaroni and cheese—maybe better than Mom's—that will become a family favorite.

SERVES: 8-10
RECOMMENDED PELLETS:
Oak, Pecan, or Apple

INGREDIENTS
2 pounds elbow macaroni
12 tablespoons butter (1-1/2 sticks), plus extra for buttering the pan
1/2 cup flour
1 teaspoon dry mustard
1-1/2 to 2 cups milk
2 pounds velveeta® or american cheese, cut into 1/2-inch cubes
1-1/2 cups grated mild cheddar cheese
2 cups plain dry breadcrumbs
Salt and black pepper
Paprika
1 disposable aluminum roasting pan, or large heat-proof casserole.

DIRECTIONS
1. Bring 5 quarts of water to a boil in a large stockpot over high heat. Add 1 tablespoon of salt. Add the macaroni, and stir. Cook for 2 minutes less than the time recommended on

the package, stirring periodically to keep the pasta from sticking. The pasta will continue to cook in the Traeger. Drain well, and transfer to a large mixing bowl.

2. Meanwhile, melt 8 tablespoons (1 Stick) of butter in a medium saucepan over medium heat. Gradually add the flour and mustard, whisking constantly. Continue whisking for about 2 minutes, being careful that the mixture doesn't begin to brown. The butter/flour mixture will bubble. Gradually whisk in 1-1/2 Cups of milk; whisk continuously until the mixture is smooth. Reduce the heat to medium-low and stir in the Velveeta®, one-third at a time, until all the cheese is incorporated and melted. Add more milk if the cheese sauce seems too thick. Season to taste with salt and pepper. Pour the cheese sauce over the pasta and stir gently with a rubber spatula or wooden spoon. Butter the roasting pan or casserole. Pour the macaroni and cheese evenly into the pan. Sprinkle the Cheddar cheese on top.

3. Melt the remaining 4 tablespoons of butter in a saucepan. Add the breadcrumbs, and stir to coat with butter. Spread the breadcrumbs evenly over the top of the macaroni and cheese. Dust lightly with paprika.

4. When ready to cook, start the Traeger grill on Smoke with the lid open until the fire is established (4 to 5 minutes). Set the temperature to 350 degrees F and preheat, lid closed, for 10 to 15 minutes.

5. Bake the macaroni and cheese for 45 minutes to 1 hour, or until the mixture is hot and bubbling and the breadcrumbs are golden brown.

LOBSTER TAIL

A pair of kitchen shears—or even tin snips—will help you release the succulent lobster meat from the tough shell. Resting the lobster meat on top of the split shell while keeping it attached at the base of the tail is a popular way of presenting lobster in restaurants.

SERVES: 2
RECOMMENDED PELLETS:
Oak, Apple, Pecan

INGREDIENTS
2 lobster tails, 8 to 10 ounces each, defrosted if frozen
8 tablespoons butter
2 tablespoons fresh lemon juice
1 teaspoon paprika
1/2 teaspoon garlic salt
1/4 teaspoon freshly ground black pepper
2 tablespoons fresh parsley, chopped (optional)

DIRECTIONS

1. Prepare the lobster by cutting down the middle of the tough shell toward the tail with kitchen shears. Using your fingers, gently pry the meat from the shell, keeping it attached at the base of the tail. Lift the meat so it is resting on top of the split shell (again, keeping it atttached at the base of the tail). Make a slit down the middle of the meat.

Place the lobster tails on a rimmed baking sheet.

2. Melt the butter in a small saucepan over medium-low heat. Whisk in the lemon juice, paprika, garlic salt, pepper, and parsley (if using). Pour about 1 tablespoon of the butter mixture over each lobster tail. Keep the remaining butter mixture warm.

3. When ready to cook, start the Traeger grill on Smoke with the lid open until the fire is established (4 to 5 minutes). Set the temperature to 400 degrees F and preheat, lid closed, for 10 to 15 minutes.

4. Remove the lobster tails from the baking sheet and arrange them directly on the grill grate. Cook for 25 to 30 minutes, or until the meat is white and opaque. Transfer the lobster tails to a platter or plates. Serve with the reserved butter mixture.

STEAKHOUSE-STYLE BAKED POTATOES

For an inexpensive but festive weeknight supper, set up a "potato bar" with baked potatoes and any accompaniments your family likes, from bacon bits to sliced pickled jalapenos. If you prefer a more toothsome skin on your baked potato, do not wrap it in foil.

SERVES: 4
RECOMMENDED PELLETS:
Hickory, Oak, Pecan, Mesquite

INGREDIENTS
4 extra-large baking potatoes, such as Idaho
2 tablespoons extra- virgin olive oil or vegetable oil
Traeger Beef Rub, or coarse salt (such as kosher or sea) and coarsely ground black pepper
Butter
Sour cream
Fresh chives or scallions (green onions), trimmed and thinly sliced (optional)

DIRECTIONS
1. Scrub the outside of the potatoes thoroughly under cold running water with a vegetable brush. Dry with paper towels. Rub the oil over each potato, season very generously with the Traeger Beef Rub, and wrap in aluminum foil.

2. When ready to cook, start the Traeger grill on Smoke with the lid open until the fire is established (4 to 5 minutes). Set the temperature to 400 degrees F and preheat, lid closed, for 10 to 15 minutes.

3. Arrange the potatoes directly on the grill grate and bake until tender, about 1 to 1-1/4 hours. (To test for doneness, run a skewer or knife through the center of a potato: It should go through without any resistance.) Transfer the potatoes to a platter or plates. Using a sharp knife, cut a lengthwise slit in each to let the steam escape. Squeeze the narrow ends of the potato to "fluff" it up.

Serve immediately with butter, sour cream, and chives.

SMOKED PORTOBELLO MUSHROOM "BURGERS"

Meaty-tasting Portobello mushrooms, marinated, infused with wood smoke, and topped with grilled onions and cheese, will not only please any vegetarians at your table—the carnivores will be satisfied, too. Whether you practice "Meatless Mondays" or not, give these a try.

SERVES: 4
RECOMMENDED PELLETS:
Any

INGREDIENTS
4 large portobello mushrooms, each 4- to 5-inches across
3/4 cup Traeger Carne Asada Marinade, or your favorite marinade for beef
1 onion, peeled and sliced into 1/2-inch rounds
4 ounces mozzarella or muenster cheese, thinly sliced
1 large ripe tomato, thinly sliced
4 tablespoons butter, melted
4 large kaiser-style hamburger rolls, split
1 large ripe tomato, thinly sliced
Pickles, lettuce leaves, mayonnaise, mustard, and ketchup for serving

DIRECTIONS

1. Wipe the mushroom caps clean with a damp paper towel. Remove the stems. Put the mushrooms and the onion slices into a resealable bag along with the Traeger Carne Asada Marinade. Let marinate, refrigerated, for 4 to 6 hours. Drain. You can refrigerate the marinade and reuse if desired, since it only touched vegetables, and not meat.

2. When ready to cook, start the Traeger grill on Smoke with the lid open until the fire is established (4 to 5 minutes).

3. Arrange the mushrooms (gill-side down) and onion slices on the grill grate and smoke for 30 minutes. Increase the temperature to 350 degrees F, and flip the mushrooms gill-side up. Cook the mushrooms and onions for 15 to 20 minutes more, or until the mushrooms are tender. The onions can still retain a bit of crunch. When the mushrooms are almost done, top each with one-fourth of the cheese. Brush the cut sides of the rolls with the melted butter. Grill, cut-side down, for a few minutes, or until they just begin to brown.

4. Transfer the bottom halves of the buns to plates or a platter. Top with the cheese- filled mushroom, onion slices, tomato, pickle, lettuce leaves, and bun tops. Serve with the suggested condiments

CLASSIC GREEN BEAN CASSEROLE

The Campbell's Soup Company scored a hit when they introduced Americans to this casserole in 1955. We've seen versions that use homemade cream of mushroom soup and even French-fried shallots in lieu of the traditional crispy onion topping. But there are some things you just shouldn't mess with.

SERVES: 4
RECOMMENDED PELLETS:
Pecan

INGREDIENTS
16-ounce cans green beans, drained, or 1-1/2 pounds fresh green beans, trimmed and cooked until tender
10-3/4 ounce can cream of mushroom condensed soup
1/2 cup milk
2 teaspoons soy sauce
1/2 teaspoon worcestershire sauce
1/2 teaspoon freshly ground black pepper
1-1/3 cups french-fried onions, divided use
1/4 cup finely diced red bell pepper or jarred pimentos (optional)

DIRECTIONS

1. In a mixing bowl, combine the beans, soup, milk, soy sauce, Worcestershire sauce, black pepper, 2/3 cup of the onions, and red pepper, if using. Transfer to a 11/2 quart casserole dish.

2. When ready to cook, start the Traeger grill on Smoke with the lid open until the fire is established (4 to 5 minutes). Set the temperature to 350 degrees F and preheat, lid closed, for 10 to 15 minutes.

3. Cook the casserole until the filling is hot and bubbling, 35 to 40 minutes. Top with the remaining onions and cook for 5 to 10 minutes more, or until the onions are crisp and beginning to brown.

JALAPENO POPPERS

These are always popular at parties. For something different, add 1/2 cup diced shrimp or crabmeat to the cheese mixture.

SERVES: 8
RECOMMENDED PELLETS:
Hickory, Mesquite, Oak

INGREDIENTS
18 medium to large jalapeno peppers
8 ounces cream cheese, at room temperature
4 ounces grated mexican four-cheese blend or cheddar cheese
1 teaspoon chili powder, or more to taste
1/2 teaspoon garlic salt
2 scallions (green onions), trimmed, white and green parts minced

8 to 10 slices of thin-cut bacon

DIRECTIONS

1. Cut each jalapeno in half lengthwise and remove the ribs and seeds. A baby spoon or demitasse spoon works well for this. (You may want to wear latex gloves.)

2. In a mixing bowl, combine the cream cheese, Mexican cheese, chili powder, and garlic salt until well-blended. Stir in the scallions. Transfer the mixture to a quart-size resealable plastic bag. With a scissors, clip about 1/2-INCh off one of the lower corners to make a pastry bag. Squeeze the cheese mixture into the jalapeno pepper halves. (Leftover cheese mixture is wonderful on baked potatoes.) Cut the bacon crosswise into pieces long enough to wrap around the middle of each jalapeno, seam-side down. Arrange on a baking sheet covered with foil or parchment paper.

3. When ready to cook, start the Traeger grill on Smoke with the lid open until the fire is established (4 to 5 minutes). Set the temperature to 350 degrees F and preheat, lid closed, for 10 to 15 minutes.

4. Roast the jalapenos for 30 minutes, or until the peppers have softened, the bacon is cooked, and the cheese is hot and bubbling. Let cool for a few minutes before serving.

SMOKED SALMON

A short romp in vodka or other spirits (rum, gin, whiskey, etc.) mutes any fishiness in the salmon, and adds subtle flavor to this fully cooked, hot- smoked fillet. It's great for breakfast with bagels and cream cheese, or even folded into scrambled eggs or tucked into an omelet. But it can double as an appetizer, too, especially when served with the traditional accompaniments of chopped hard-cooked egg, diced onion, and capers.

SERVES: 6

RECOMMENDED PELLETS:
Alder, Apple, Cherry

INGREDIENTS
1 salmon fillet (1-1/2 to 2 pounds), preferably wild-caught
1 cup vodka or apple juice
1 cup brown sugar or brown sugar substitute, such as splenda®
1/2 cup coarse (kosher) salt
1 tablespoon coarse black pepper

DIRECTIONS

1. Run your fingers over the salmon fillet and remove any pin bones you find with kitchen tweezers or needle-nose pliers. Put the salmon fillet in a large resealable plastic bag and pour the vodka over it. Massage the bag to make sure the salmon is immersed, then refrigerate for 1 to 2 hours.

2. Make the cure: Combine the sugar, salt, and black pepper in another large resealable plastic bag. Drain the fish. Discard the vodka. Add the fillet to the sugar mixture, making sure the salmon is thoroughly coated. Refrig- erate for 2 to 4 hours.

3. Rinse the cure off the salmon and dry with paper towels.

4. When ready to cook, start the Traeger grill on Smoke with the lid open until the fire is established (4 to 5 minutes).

5. Arrange the salmon (skin-side down, if it has skin) on the grill grate. Smoke for 30 min- utes. Increase the temperature to 225 degrees F. Cook the salmon for 45 minutes to an hour, or until the fish flakes easily with a fork. (The exact time will depend on the thickness of the fillet.) There is no need to turn the fish. Using a large thin spatula, transfer the salmon to a wire rack to cool. Cover the fish with plastic wrap and refrigerate until serving time. Can be made 2 to 3 days ahead.

TRAEGER HOT SMOKED TROUT

Trout smoked on your Traeger and served as an appetizer is guaranteed to impress dinner guests. It's terrific when served with pickled onions on cocktail breads, but can be "stretched" by mixing a cup of flaked smoked trout with 8 ounces of room temperature cream cheese, 3 tablespoons of softened butter, 1 tablespoon of fresh lemon juice, salt and pepper to taste, and a few drops of hot sauce. Minced red onion, scallions, or chives are a nice addition, too.

SERVES: 4-6
RECOMMENDED PELLETS:
Alder, Hickory, Oak

INGREDIENTS
1/2 cup brown sugar
1/4 cup kosher salt
1 tablespoon pickling spice
1 quart cold water
1-1/2 pounds trout (3 to 4), cleaned and butterflied, skin-on

DIRECTIONS
1. Make the brine: Combine the brown sugar, salt, pickling spice, and water in a large pitcher or canning jar. Stir until the sugar and salt crystals dissolve. Open the trout. Run your fingers over the flesh to detect bones; remove any you find with kitchen tweezers or needle-nose pliers. Submerge the trout in the brine; refrigerate for 2 to 3 hours, but no longer.

2. When ready to cook, start the Traeger grill on Smoke with the lid open until the fire is established (4 to 5 minutes). Close the lid.

3. Remove the trout from the brine, knock off any large pieces of the pickling spices, and dry the fish on paper towels. Arrange the trout skin-side down on the grill grate.
Smoke for 30 to 40 minutes until the flesh turns opaque and flakes easily when prodded with a finger or fork. Transfer to a cooling rack. When cool, cover with plastic wrap and refrigerate until serving time. Smoked trout will keep, refrigerated, for 2 to 3 days.

CHICKEN QUESADILLAS

Beloved as an after-school-snack, quesadillas are also a great way to kick off a backyard party! Assemble these grill-side and serve hot as your guests arrive. Leave the chicken out for a vegetarian option.

SERVES: 4-6
RECOMMENDED PELLETS:
Any

INGREDIENTS
4 10-inch flour tortillas
vegetable oil
2 cups grated monterey jack or pepper jack cheese
2 cups shredded or chopped cooked chicken (preferably made at a previous grill session)

1 small bunch fresh cilantro, leaves pulled off stems
2 medium tomatoes, seeded and diced
4 scallions (green onions), trimmed, green and white parts thinly sliced
1/4 cup pickled jalapeno slices, chopped (optional)
salt
salsa and/or sour cream for serving

DIRECTIONS

1. Lay a tortilla down on a rimmed baking sheet (or a large piece of aluminum foil) coated lightly with vegetable oil. Leave one- half of the tortilla bare. Top the other half with some of the cheese, chicken, cilantro leaves, tomatoes, scallions, and pickled jalapenos, if desired. Season with salt. Finish with a little more grated cheese. (This will "glue" the other ingredients together as it melts.) Fold the bare half of the tortilla over the filled half and set aside. Repeat the process with the remaining tortillas.

2. When ready to cook, start the Traeger grill on Smoke with the lid open until the fire is established (4 to 5 minutes). Set the tempera- ture to 375 degrees F and preheat, lid closed, for 10 to 15 minutes.

3. With a large spatula, carefully transfer the quesadillas to the grill grate. Cook until the cheese is melted and the outside is begin- ning to brown (8 to 10 minutes total). Using the spatula, turn once half- way through the cooking time. Cut each quesadilla into three wedges with a scissors or sharp knife. Serve with salsa and/or sour cream.

TRAEGER SAUSAGE "FATTY"

Popular for several years with barbecue and smoking enthusiasts, "fatties" are usually 1-pound logs of smoked breakfast-type sausage (sometimes known as chubs). Not only are they wonderful served with eggs, biscuits, or French toast, but when thinly sliced, they can double as appetizers. A bit of ground coffee added to the rub echoes the breakfast theme. If you're smoking one, you might as well smoke two. They'll disappear quickly. By the way, when you slice the sausage, you'll see a lovely pink smoke ring near the surface—a barbecuer's "badge of honor".

SERVES: 4
RECOMMENDED PELLETS:
Hickory, Oak, Alder, Pecan

INGREDIENTS
1 1-pound uncooked sausage chub, such as Bob Evans or Jimmy
Dean brands, any flavor
Traeger Pork and Poultry Rub, or your favorite barbecue rub
1 tablespoon fine- to medium-grind coffee

DIRECTIONS
1. Carefully remove the plastic wrapping from the sausage so the sausage remains log-shaped, about 2-1/2 to 3 inches in diameter. Season evenly with the Traeger Pork and Poultry Rub, then dust with the coffee.

2. When ready to cook, start the Traeger grill on Smoke with the lid open until the fire is established (4 to 5 minutes).

Smoke the sausage for 1 hour. Increase the heat to 225 degrees F. Continue to cook the sausage until an instant-read meat thermometer inserted through the end reads 160 degrees F, about 45 minutes to an hour. Let rest for 15 minutes before slicing. If you can wait that long!

GRILLED SHRIMP COCKTAIL

In our estimation, grilled shrimp is far superior to boiled shrimp in this American classic.

SERVES: 8

RECOMMENDED PELLETS:
Pecan, Apple

INGREDIENTS
2 pounds jumbo or extra-jumbo shrimp (about 36), peeled and deveined, tail-on
1/4 cup extra-virgin olive oil
Traeger veggie shake, or your favorite barbecue rub
1 cup traeger chili sauce, or your favorite chili sauce
2 tablespoons prepared horseradish, or more to taste
1 tablespoon fresh lemon or lime juice
1 teaspoon worcestershire sauce
A few drops of tabasco® sauce
Freshly ground black pepper
Lemon wedges for serving
6-inch bamboo skewers

DIRECTIONS

1. In a medium bowl, toss the shrimp to coat with the olive oil and about 2 teaspoons of Traeger Veggie Shake. Thread the shrimp on the bamboo skewers. Combine the chili sauce, horseradish, lemon juice, Worcestershire sauce, and Tabasco® sauce in a small bowl, whisking to blend. Season to taste with pepper.

2. When ready to cook, start the Traeger grill on Smoke with the lid open until the fire is established (4 to 5 minutes). Set the temperature to 450 degrees F (High) and preheat, lid closed, for 10 to 15 minutes.

3. Arrange the shrimp skewers on the grill grate. Grill until firm and opaque, 2 to 4 minutes per side. Arrange on a plate or platter with the sauce and lemon wedges.

BARBECUED CHICKEN NACHOS

Have you ever ordered a plate of nachos in a restaurant, only to discover many of the chips missed out on the toppings? Not only is this recipe a twist on traditional versions, but each chip carries a payload of all the ingredients.

SERVES: 4
RECOMMENDED PELLETS:
Apple, Hickory
INGREDIENTS
1-1/4 pounds boneless skinless chicken breasts
Traeger pork and poultry rub, or taco seasoning
1/2 to 3/4 cup traeger regular barbecue sauce
24 large tortilla chips (not broken)
3 cups (12 ounces) grated mexican four- cheese blend
1/2 cup sliced black olives, drained
Sliced pickled jalapenos (optional)
3 scallions (green onions), trimmed, white and green parts thinly sliced
1 cup sour cream, for serving

DIRECTIONS

1. Season the chicken breasts with the temperature to 350 degrees F and preheat, lid closed, for 10 to 15 minutes. Traeger Pork and Poultry Rub.

2. When ready to cook, start the Traeger grill on Smoke with the lid open until the fire is established (4 to 5 minutes). Set the

3. Arrange the chicken breasts on the grill grate and cook, turning once halfway through the cooking time, for 25 to 30 minutes, or until the internal temperature when read on an instant-read meat thermometer is 170 degrees F. Transfer to a cutting board and let rest for 3 minutes. Leave the grill on if you are making the nachos immediately.

4. Dice the chicken into small cubes, 1/2-INCh or less. Transfer to a mixing bowl and pour 1/2 Cup of Traeger Regular Barbecue Sauce over the diced chicken. Stir gently to coat each piece. (Add more sauce if needed, but not so much that the mixture is "gloppy".) Set aside, or cover and refrigerate if not making the nachos immediately.

5. Lay the tortilla chips in a single layer on a rimmed baking sheet or pizza pan. Sprinkle evenly with half the cheese. Spoon a little of the barbecued chicken mixture on each chip. Top with black olives and pickled jalapeno, if desired. Sprinkle the remaining half of the cheese evenly over the chips. Scatter the sliced onions over the chips.

6. Put the baking sheet on the grill grate. Bake until the chips are crisp and the cheese is melted, 12 to 15 minutes. With a spatula, transfer the nachos to a plate or platter. Serve immediately with the sour cream.

GRILLED CORN SALSA

Salsa...it's not just for chips anymore. Grilled Corn Salsa is so versatile, you can serve it over grilled chicken, beef, or steak fish like tuna, halibut, or swordfish. Or pair it with grilled shrimp for a unique shrimp cocktail. Vary the salsa by adding diced red bell pepper or avocado, or a can of black beans, rinsed and drained.

SERVES: 6-8
RECOMMENDED PELLETS:
Hickory, Mesquite

INGREDIENTS
4 tomatoes, such as Roma, halved
1 medium-size onion, peeled and quartered through the root end
1/2 to 2 jalapeno peppers, or more to taste, halved
3 ears sweet corn, husked
2 Cloves garlic, finely minced
1 to 2 tablespoons vegetable oil
Fresh lime juice to taste
1-1/2 teaspoons Traeger Veggie Shake, or salt and freshly ground pepper to taste

1 teaspoon cumin
1/4 cup fresh cilantro leaves, chopped

DIRECTIONS

1. When ready to cook, start the Traeger grill on Smoke with the lid open until the fire is established (4 to 5 minutes). Set the temperature to 450 degrees F (High) and preheat, lid closed, for 10 to 15 minutes.

2. Arrange the tomatoes, onion, and jalapeno(s) cut-sides down, on the grill grate. Grill until the vegetables have nice char marks on the cut sides. Grill the corn at the same time, turning frequently, until some of the kernels are deeply browned.

3. Transfer the vegetables to a cutting board and let cool. With a sharp knife, cut the corn kernels off the cob (if you work on a damp towel the kernels won't scatter so much).
Slip the skins off the tomatoes and dice. Dice the onion. Seed the jalapenos (or leave the seeds in for a noticeably hotter salsa), and mince. Transfer the grilled vegetables to a mixing bowl. Stir in the garlic, vegetable oil, lime juice, Traeger Veggie Shake, cumin, and cilantro. Serve at room temperature for the best flavor. The salsa can be made several hours ahead, but is best the day it is made. Refrigerate any leftovers in a covered container.

PEPPERONI-PROVOLONE BREAD

Highly addictive as an appetizer or accompaniment to an Italian dinner.

SERVES: 8
RECOMMENDED PELLETS:
Oak, Apple, Pecan

INGREDIENTS
1 loaf frozen bread dough, such as Rhodes
Extra-virgin olive oil
1 teaspoon dried oregano
1 teaspoon dried basil
1 teaspoon dried parsley
4 ounces thinly sliced pepperoni
4 ounces thinly sliced provolone cheese, or mozzarella
Cornmeal for dusting the baking sheet

DIRECTIONS

1. Thaw the bread dough and let it rise ac-cording to the package directions. On a lightly floured kitchen counter or other flat surface, roll and stretch the dough into a 12- by 18-inch rectangle. (This takes a little patience if the dough is very elastic. Let it rest for a few minutes and try again.) Brush with olive oil, and sprinkle evenly with half of the oregano, basil, and parsley. Arrange the pepperoni in a single layer on the dough, leaving a 1-INCh border on all sides. Lay the cheese on top of the pepperoni. Starting on the long side, roll the dough up evenly jelly roll-style. Pinch the long seam together along its length. Pinch the ends together and tuck under the loaf, crimping the dough to keep the cheese and pepperoni enclosed.

2. Lay the bread, seam-side down, on an oiled baking sheet dusted lightly with cornmeal.
Brush the top and sides with olive oil, and sprinkle the remaining dried herbs evenly over it. Using a bread knife, slice shallow vents in the top on a diagonal. Cover with oiled plastic wrap and let rise in a warm place for 30 minutes.

4. When ready to cook, start the Traeger grill on Smoke with the lid open until the fire is established (4 to 5 minutes). Set the tempera- ture to 350 degrees F and preheat, lid closed, for 10 to 15 minutes.

CPSIA information can be obtained
at www.ICGtesting.com
Printed in the USA
LVHW020234040121
675399LV00001B/53

5. Remove the plastic wrap from the bread. Transfer the baking sheet with the bread to the grill. Bake for 40 to 50 minutes, or until the bread is brown and baked through. (It's better to overbake than underbake, in this case.) Let the bread cool completely on a rack before slicing and serving.

DIRECTIONS

1. Thaw the bread dough and let it rise ac-cording to the package directions. On a lightly floured kitchen counter or other flat surface, roll and stretch the dough into a 12- by 18-inch rectangle. (This takes a little patience if the dough is very elastic. Let it rest for a few minutes and try again.) Brush with olive oil, and sprinkle evenly with half of the oregano, basil, and parsley. Arrange the pepperoni in a single layer on the dough, leaving a 1-INCh border on all sides. Lay the cheese on top of the pepperoni. Starting on the long side, roll the dough up evenly jelly roll-style. Pinch the long seam together along its length. Pinch the ends together and tuck under the loaf, crimping the dough to keep the cheese and pepperoni enclosed.

2. Lay the bread, seam-side down, on an oiled baking sheet dusted lightly with cornmeal.
Brush the top and sides with olive oil, and sprinkle the remaining dried herbs evenly over it. Using a bread knife, slice shallow vents in the top on a diagonal. Cover with oiled plastic wrap and let rise in a warm place for 30 minutes.

4. When ready to cook, start the Traeger grill on Smoke with the lid open until the fire is established (4 to 5 minutes). Set the tempera- ture to 350 degrees F and preheat, lid closed, for 10 to 15 minutes.

5. Remove the plastic wrap from the bread. Transfer the baking sheet with the bread to the grill. Bake for 40 to 50 minutes, or until the bread is brown and baked through. (It's better to overbake than underbake, in this case.) Let the bread cool completely on a rack before slicing and serving.

CPSIA information can be obtained
at www.ICGtesting.com
Printed in the USA
LVHW020234040121
675399LV00001B/53